Water, Race, and Disease

NBER Series on Long-term Factors in Economic Development
A National Bureau of Economic Research Series
Edited by Claudia Goldin

Also in the series

Claudia Goldin, *Understanding the Gender Gap: An Economic History of American Women* (Oxford University Press, 1990)

Roderick Floud, Kenneth Wachter, and Annabel Gregory, *Height, Health and History: Nutritional Status in the United Kingdom, 1750–1980* (Cambridge University Press, 1990)

Robert A. Margo, *Race and Schooling in the South, 1880–1950: An Economic History* (University of Chicago Press, 1990)

Samuel H. Preston and Michael R. Haines, *Fatal Years: Child Mortality in Late Nineteenth-Century America* (Princeton University Press, 1991)

Barry Eichengreen, *Golden Fetters: The Gold Standard and the Great Depression, 1919–1939* (Oxford University Press, 1992)

Ronald N. Johnson and Gary D. Libecap, *The Federal Civil Service System and the Problem of Bureaucracy: The Economics and Politics of Institutional Change* (University of Chicago Press, 1994)

Naomi R. Lamoreaux, *Insider Lending: Banks, Personal Connections, and Economic Development in Industrial New England, 1784–1912* (Cambridge University Press, 1994)

Lance E. Davis, Robert E. Gallman, and Karin Gleiter, *In Pursuit of Leviathan: Technology, Institutions, Productivity, and Profits in American Whaling, 1816–1906* (University of Chicago Press, 1997)

Dora L. Costa, *The Evolution of Retirement: An American Economic History, 1880–1990* (University of Chicago Press, 1998)

Joseph P. Ferrie, *Yankeys Now: Immigrants in the Antebellum U.S., 1840–1860* (Oxford University Press, 1999)

Robert A. Margo, *Wages and Labor Markets in the United States, 1820–1860* (University of Chicago Press, 2000)

Price V. Fishback and Shawn Everett Kantor, *A Prelude to the Welfare State: The Origins of Workers' Compensation* (University of Chicago Press, 2000)

Gerardo della Paolera and Alan M. Taylor, *Straining at the Anchor: The Argentine Currency Board and the Search for Macroeconomic Stability, 1880–1935* (University of Chicago Press, 2001)

Water, Race, and Disease

Werner Troesken

The MIT Press
Cambridge, Massachusetts
London, England

This book was set in Palatino on 3B2 by Asco Typesetters, Hong Kong.
Printed and bound in the United States of America.

Library of Congress Cataloging-in-Publication Data

Troesken, Werner, 1963–
  Water, race, and disease / Werner Troesken.
    p.   cm. — (NBER series on long-term factors in economic development)
  Includes bibliographical references and index.
  ISBN 0-262-20148-8 (hbk. : alk. paper)
    1. African Americans—Health and hygiene—History. 2. African Americans—Social conditions—History. 3. Waterborne infection—Prevention—United States—History. 4. Health and race—United States—History. I. Title. II. Series.
  RA448.5.N4T76   2004
  362.1′089′96073—dc22   2003065135

10 9 8 7 6 5 4 3 2 1

To Nolan, Rick, and Sara,
for a year of great conversations.

Contents

Relation of the Directors to the Work and Publications of the NBER

1. The object of the NBER is to ascertain and present to the economics profession, and to the public more generally, important economic facts and their interpretation in a scientific manner without policy recommendations. The Board of Directors is charged with the responsibility of ensuring that the work of the NBER is carried on in strict conformity with this object.

2. The President shall establish an internal review process to ensure that book manuscripts proposed for publication DO NOT contain policy recommendations. This shall apply both to the proceedings of conferences and to manuscripts by a single author or by one or more co-authors but shall not apply to authors of comments at NBER conferences who are not NBER affiliates.

3. No book manuscript reporting research shall be published by the NBER until the President has sent to each member of the Board a notice that a manuscript is recommended for publication and that in the President's opinion it is suitable for publication in accordance with the above principles of the NBER. Such notification will include a table of contents and an abstract or summary of the manuscript's content, a list of contributors if applicable, and a response form for use by Directors who desire a copy of the manuscript for review. Each manuscript shall contain a summary drawing attention to the nature and treatment of the problem studied and the main conclusions reached.

4. No volume shall be published until forty-five days have elapsed from the above notification of intention to publish it. During this period a copy shall be sent to any Director requesting it, and if any Director objects to publication on the grounds that the manuscript contains policy recommendations, the objection will be presented to the author(s) or editor(s). In case of dispute, all members of the Board shall be notified, and the President shall appoint an ad hoc committee of the Board to decide the matter; thirty days additional shall be granted for this purpose.

5. The President shall present annually to the Board a report describing the internal manuscript review process, any objections made by Directors before publication or by anyone after publication, any disputes about such matters, and how they were handled.

6. Publications of the NBER issued for informational purposes concerning the work of the Bureau, or issued to inform the public of the activities at the Bureau, including but not limited to the NBER Digest and Reporter, shall be consistent with the object stated in paragraph 1. They shall contain a specific disclaimer noting that they have not passed through the review procedures required in this resolution. The Executive Committee of the Board is charged with the review of all such publications from time to time.

7. NBER working papers and manuscripts distributed on the Bureau's web site are not deemed to be publications for the purpose of this resolution, but they shall be consistent with the object stated in paragraph 1. Working papers shall contain a specific disclaimer noting that they have not passed through the review procedures required in this resolution. The NBER's web site shall contain a similar disclaimer. The President shall establish an internal review process to ensure that the working papers and the web site do not contain policy recommendations, and shall report annually to the Board on this process and any concerns raised in connection with it.

8. Unless otherwise determined by the Board or exempted by the terms of paragraphs 6 and 7, a copy of this resolution shall be printed in each NBER publication as described in paragraph 2 above.

Acknowledgments

For reading and commenting on the entire book manuscript, I thank Todd Bridges, Dora Costa, Claudia Goldin, Bob Margo, John Murray, Daniel Scott Smith, and Melissa Thomasson. For commenting on specific chapters or related papers, I thank Patty Beeson, Peter Blanck, Lou Cain, Bill Collins, Sara Ellison, Price Fishback, Robert Fogel, Rick Geddes, Maurine Greenwald, Mike Haines, Ed Lazear, Nolan McCarty, Ken Sokoloff, Joel Tarr, Jeff Williamson, and Gavin Wright. I thank Nancy Tannery for locating a number of useful articles on typhoid fever, and the beach group for helping with the title. Parts of this book and related papers have also been presented at the following universities and conferences, and I thank the participants for their thoughts and suggestions: UC-Berkeley, UCLA, Chicago, the annual meetings of the Cliometrics Society, Columbia, the DC-Area Economic History Workshop, Harvard, the Hoover Institution, Miami University (Ohio), Montana State, Ohio State, Pittsburgh, the annual meetings of the Social Science History Association, and Stanford.

The research for this book has been funded in part by a grant from the NIH/NIA, AG10120-09A1, 2001–2006, which is gratefully acknowledged. The research for this book was started while I was a National Fellow at the Hoover Institution, and I thank Hoover for providing such a wonderful intellectual environment. I also thank Cambridge University Press for allowing me to reprint portions of my article, "The Limits of Jim Crow: Race and the Provision of Public Water and Sewer in American Cities, 1880–1925," which appeared in the *Journal of Economic History*, volume 62, no. 3 (September 2002), pp. 734–72. Finally, I thank the editorial staff at MIT Press and Susan Jones for their suggestions and attention to detail. Of course, I retain sole responsibility for all remaining errors.

Preface

In 1900, public health officials in the United States wanted to separate privies and wells. They were particularly concerned about separating black privies from white wells because in a world run by racists, the most important kind of separation was the separation of the races. To die from typhoid was one thing. To die from typhoid one caught by drinking water tainted with the wastes of a black man's privy was quite another. Ironically, the best way to separate black privies and white wells, and to reduce typhoid, was through integration. Integrating the services supplied to the races so that they were all part of one large system of water and sewer mains solved the problem. When towns finished building their water and sewer systems, typhoid disappeared.

It was not only typhoid that drove cities to integrate their infrastructures, it was also the geography of race, a geography that seems peculiar to us today. In 1900, urban blacks and whites, particularly those in the South, lived together, almost side by side. Blacks lived on one block, whites on the next. Whites lived on the main street, blacks in an alley or on a small side street just off the main thoroughfare. There was no single "black side" of town. There were many black areas distributed throughout the town. In this intimate setting, race really mattered. And so did the relative aesthetics of sewers and privies. The stench of another white man's privy was one thing; the stench of a black man's privy was quite another.

In developing this line of argument, I am attributing something new to the racist ideologies that dominated American thought and practice during the nineteenth and early twentieth centuries. We usually think of these ideologies as causing public officials to deny service, or at best provide inadequate service, to African Americans—segregated public schools come immediately to mind. Water and sewer services were an exception to this pattern of denial. Racism did not undermine the case for bringing public water and sewer services to African-American homes; it strengthened it.

However, the larger story here is not about ideology. It is about African-American life, and about how it has improved over the course of the past century. Consider, for example, the 40-year span from 1900 to 1940. This period witnessed tremendous improvements in life expectancy among urban blacks, both in absolute terms and relative to whites. These improvements were not limited to a particular region or set of cities; they were pervasive. If one contemplates the time and place in which these improvements occurred, they are remarkable. How is it that during this time—probably the peak of Jim Crow—such improvements could have occurred? The story here is mostly about answering this question and others like it. How and why the ideology of race pushed cities to install water and sewer lines in black neighborhoods helps answer such demographic questions and is part of the larger story, but in that sense the role of ideology is secondary.

In making the case for this story, I build on the insights of scholars from many disciplines, including demography, economics, geography, history, law, and medicine. For example, recent research in demography and medicine demonstrates that exposure to typhoid at an early stage in life significantly increases the probability of heart problems later in life. This finding helps establish the argument in chapter 2 that building water and sewer systems not only reduced waterborne disease rates, it also promoted better overall health and reduced mortality from nonwaterborne diseases. Similarly, research in geography shows that cities were much less segregated in 1890 and 1900 than they are today. This finding helps establish the book's larger argument about the difficulties of denying African-American neighborhoods public water and sewer lines.

I have also tried to draw from as many independent sources of evidence as possible. For example, the qualitative evidence I present ranges from a historical analysis of the case law on discrimination in the provision of municipal services, to maps that reconstruct the location of black and white households in relation to water and sewer lines. The quantitative evidence I present ranges from statistical tests that explore how black and white waterborne disease rates responded to improvements in local water and sewer systems, to an examination of a data set that includes some quarter of a million households and contains information on household access to public water and sewer lines. I also make use of data from the Negro Mortality Project, a hitherto unexploited source. Conducted under the auspices of black leaders in 1897, the Negro Mortality Project was an ambitious census-like survey of more than a thousand urban-dwelling African-American households. Although each of these sources of evidence is subject to its own set of concerns and potential biases, they all point toward the same conclusion. There was much less discrimination in the provision of public water and sewer services than one might otherwise expect given the time and place.

Water, Race, and Disease

1   Introduction

1.1   The Puzzling History of African-American Mortality

The Civil Rights movement was a watershed event in American history. In the words of the economic-historian Gavin Wright, the movement was a "revolution," an event that not only improved the economic and political lives of millions of individuals, but an event that changed in fundamental ways the nature of an entire region. Like the British antislavery movement and the collapse of Soviet communism, the Civil Rights movement transformed a society from the bottom to the top. There was political advancement. The proportion of the African-American population registered to vote doubled, increasing from less than 30 percent in 1960 to 60 percent in 1970. There was also economic advancement. Wages and occupational mobility for African Americans increased dramatically as a result of the passage of the Civil Rights Act and the creation of the Equal Employment Opportunity Commission (EEOC). This was particularly true in the American South where during the 1960s, the black-white wage deficit was nearly cut in half, and well-paying jobs once reserved for whites became available to blacks. Similar improvements can be documented in terms of educational funding, rates of educational enrollment and literacy, access to housing and credit, incidence of poverty and crime, and a host of other indicators of overall social and material well-being.[1]

There was, however, at least one exception to this general pattern of improvement. The civil rights era witnessed almost no improvement in African-American life expectancy, in either absolute terms or relative to whites. This can be seen in figure 1.1, which plots black and white life expectancies from 1900 to 2000. Whether one looks at the entire population or focuses exclusively on individuals living in urban areas, figure 1.1 suggests that black life expectancy did not change during the

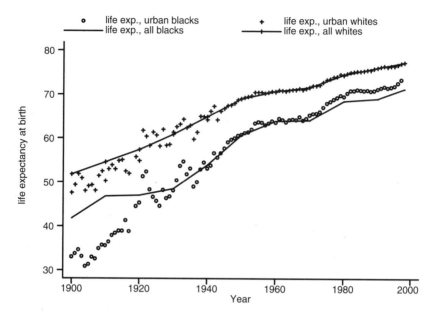

Figure 1.1
Life expectancies for black and white Americans, 1900–2000. As a measure of the lon-
gevity of urban-dwelling blacks and whites, I use data constructed by Michael Haines.
Using the original Death Registration Area (DRA) as defined by the census in 1900,
Haines estimates the life expectancy in this area from 1900 through 1998. The original
DRA was heavily skewed toward urban areas, and therefore provides a rough measure
of mortality trends in urban areas. About 82 percent of the black and 67 percent of the
white population included in the original DRA was urban, while 20 percent of the entire
black population and 43 percent of the white lived in urban areas. See Haines, "Ethnic
Differences," especially p. 10 and table 8. The estimates constructed by Haines are preferable to those reported in the *Historical Statistics* of the U.S. Census Bureau and similar
sources because in those sources the DRA changes over time. As a measure of longevity
of the entire black and white populations, I again use data from Haines and these data
cover the whole U.S. population. See Haines, "Ethnic Differences," table 3. These estimates are based on samples from the whole U.S. Census and are built following the same
general methods as employed by Preston and Haines in *Fatal Years*. However it should be
noted that Haines does not share my sanguine interpretation of his data. See Haines,
"Ethnic Differences," pp. 9–11. Source: Haines "Ethnic Differences," tables 3 (entire population) and 8 (urban population).

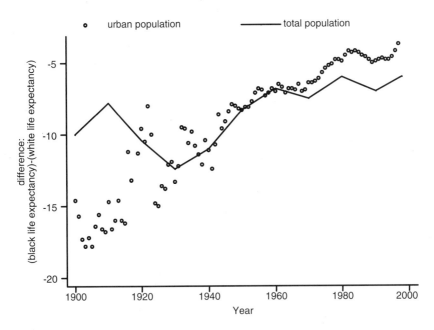

Figure 1.2
Difference between black and white life expectancies, 1900–2000. See notes to figure 1.1.
Source: Haines, "Ethnic Differences," tables 3 and 8.

1960s and rose only slightly during the 1970s. Surprisingly, the largest increases in African-American life expectancy occurred before 1950. This was particularly true for urban-dwelling blacks, who saw their life expectancy at birth rise by nearly 50 percent, from 30 years in 1900 to 44 in 1940. The rate of improvement in black life expectancy slowed after 1960, so that between 1960 and 2000 black life expectancy increased by less than 10 years. It is also notable and important that regardless of time period, urban-dwelling blacks experienced much larger absolute improvements in life expectancy than their rural counterparts.[2]

If we examine black life expectancy relative to that for whites, similar patterns emerge. To show this, figure 1.2 plots the difference between black and white life expectancies. A series for urban populations is plotted alongside a series for the entire population. For the overall population, the deficit in black life expectancy remains at about 7 years after 1960. For the urban black population, the upward trend in relative improvement stagnates between 1960 and 1970 and then rises by about 5 years during the 1970s and 1980s. The largest relative

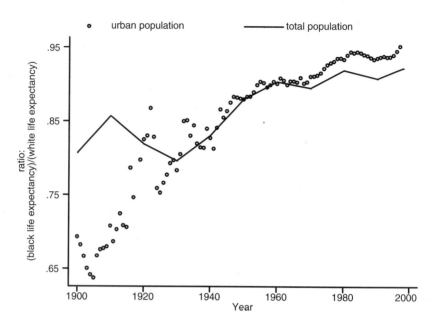

Figure 1.3
Ratio of black and white life expectancies, 1900–2000. See notes to figure 1.1. Source:
Haines, "Ethnic Differences," tables 3 and 8.

improvements in black life expectancy occurred before 1960. For the
overall population, the deficit in black life expectancy was cut in half
between 1930 and 1960, although this upward trend was preceded by
a sharp diminution in blacks' relative status between 1900 and 1930.
Urban-dwelling blacks, in contrast, experienced a steady upward trend
in their relative life expectancy between 1900 and 1960. In 1900 the life
expectancy for urban blacks was 17 years less than that for whites; by
1960, urban black life expectancy was about 7 years less than that for
whites. If one examines the ratio of black to white life expectancy, the
identical patterns emerge (see figure 1.3).

As the previous figures suggest, most of the improvement in black
life expectancy that occurred between 1900 and 1940 was concentrated
among blacks living in urban areas. Because the experience of urban-
dwelling blacks is the primary focus of this book, it is desirable to
further document and explain their mortality rates. Compare, for example, the improvements in black life expectancy that occurred in
New York, where blacks were highly urbanized, with those that occurred in North and South Carolina, where blacks lived primarily in

Table 1.1
Black and White Life Expectancy in Three States, 1920–1940

State	1920 e^0 Black	White	1940 e^0 Black	White	% Change Black	White	Absolute change Black	White
New York	38.3	53.4	54.2	64.4	0.42	0.21	15.9	11.0
North Carolina	46.6	56.7	54.4	64.4	0.17	0.14	7.8	7.7
South Carolina	44.4	55.5	51.2	64.6	0.15	0.16	6.8	9.1

Source: Ewbank, "Black Mortality."
Note: e^0 indicates life expectancy at birth.

rural areas. As table 1.1 shows, blacks in New York realized far greater gains in life expectancy, in both absolute and relative terms, than those in North and South Carolina. Black New Yorkers gained an additional 16 years of life between 1920 and 1940, while the life expectancy of blacks in the Carolinas rose only by about half that amount. It is tempting to attribute the differing experiences between New York and the Carolinas to a North/South effect. However, there is also evidence of improvement in African-American mortality when one examines crude mortality rates in southern cities. This can be seen in table 1.2, which summarizes changes in black mortality rates between 1908 and 1940 for a sample of twenty-eight cities in the American South. In all but two of these cities (Cumberland, Maryland, and Lynchburg, Virginia), black mortality rates fell between 1908 and 1940. If one examines absolute reductions in death rates, in twenty of the twenty-eight cities black death rates fell by more than white rates; if one uses percentage reductions, black rates fell by more in thirteen of these cities.[3]

These patterns are puzzling. How is it that during a time of great material and social gain (the 1960s) there was so little improvement in African-American health, while during a time of social and political deprivation (the early 1900s), there was so much improvement? More precisely, the Civil Rights movement, and the legislative changes that grew out of it, wrought tremendous improvements for African Americans economically, politically, and socially. Why did these material and social gains not manifest themselves in increased life expectancy? The rapid absolute and relative improvements in life expectancy that occurred during the early twentieth century are equally puzzling. At this time, African Americans were politically disenfranchised; racial animus was everywhere; lynchings were commonplace; schools and public facilities were segregated and black institutions were woefully

Table 1.2
Death Rates in Twenty-Eight Southern Cities: 1908–1940

City	1908 Rate Black	White	1940 Rate Black	White	% Reduction Black	White	Absolute reduction Black	White
Birmingham, Ala.	28.4	18.8	15.5	9.0	0.45	0.52	12.9	9.8
Mobile, Ala.	25.6	17.3	17.1	11.0	0.33	0.36	8.5	6.3
Montgomery, Ala.	22.3	13.7	18.6	9.5	0.17	0.31	3.7	4.2
Washington, D.C.	26.1	16.2	15.5	10.9	0.41	0.33	10.6	5.3
Jacksonville, Fla.	30.1	24.4	16.2	10.7	0.46	0.56	13.9	13.7
Atlanta, Ga.	24.8	18.7	18.8	10.1	0.24	0.46	6.0	8.6
Savannah, Ga.	26.4	15.1	20.3	11.9	0.23	0.21	6.1	3.2
Louisville, Ky.	25.3	13.9	20.2	12.1	0.20	0.13	5.1	1.8
Paducah, Ky.	21.1	13.9	19.5	10.7	0.07	0.23	1.6	3.2
New Orleans, La.	32.8	19.0	16.0	12.4	0.51	0.35	16.8	6.6
Annapolis, Md.	40.3	15.0	16.0	11.6	0.60	0.23	24.3	3.4
Baltimore, Md.	28.7	16.4	16.5	11.7	0.42	0.29	12.2	4.7
Cumberland, Md.	25.6	19.9	26.9	16.2	0.05[a]	0.19	1.3[a]	3.7
Frederick, Md.	25.0	15.4	15.9	15.2	0.36	0.01	9.1	0.2
Hagerstown, Md.	24.6	16.5	24.2	13.3	0.02	0.19	0.4	3.2
Raleigh, N.C.	25.1	29.0	16.4	11.7	0.35	0.60	8.7	17.3
Wilmington, N.C.	31.7	22.0	18.9	11.2	0.40	0.49	12.8	10.8
Charleston, S.C.	34.5	17.7	19.7	10.9	0.43	0.39	14.8	6.8
Knoxville, Tenn.	24.7	15.4	15.7	10.4	0.36	0.33	9.0	5.0
Memphis, Tenn.	18.5	15.6	14.9	9.5	0.20	0.39	3.6	6.1
Nashville, Tenn.	26.6	16.0	19.5	11.6	0.27	0.28	7.1	4.4
Galveston, Texas	23.7	15.3	16.0	14.4	0.32	0.06	7.7	0.9
Alexandria, Va.	25.3	16.7	16.2	9.6	0.36	0.43	9.1	7.1
Danville, Va.	26.3	20.5	16.7	15.8	0.37	0.23	9.6	4.7
Lynchburg, Va.	15.8	14.8	23.0	11.5	0.46[a]	0.22	7.2[a]	3.3
Norfolk, Va.	25.5	16.5	15.9	9.7	0.38	0.41	9.6	6.8
Petersburg, Va.	36.8	20.8	19.0	12.4	0.48	0.40	17.8	8.4
Richmond, Va.	30.0	18.8	16.1	10.8	0.46	0.43	13.9	8.0

Sources: U.S. Bureau of Census, *Mortality Statistics*, 1908 and 1940 volumes.
Note: Rate is total deaths per 1,000 persons.
[a] Increase in mortality.

underfunded; and while there was economic progress, the extent of that progress is subject to debate.[4] Given these obstacles, how is it that life expectancy, both in absolute terms and relative to whites, increased for urban-dwelling African Americans?

An equally important set of questions revolves around the variation in the health experiences of urban-dwelling blacks across different cities, regions, and time periods. To be more precise, the data presented earlier suggest that in the typical city there was both absolute and relative improvement in African-American life expectancy, but the same data also suggest that there was much variation around the experience of the typical city. Consider again the data presented in table 1.2. At one extreme, in Baltimore, Maryland and New Orleans, Louisiana, blacks realized absolute and relative improvements in mortality that were truly remarkable, while at the other extreme, in Cumberland and Lynchburg, black mortality rates actually worsened, in both absolute and relative terms. While the data in table 1.2 suggest that the experiences of places like Cumberland and Lynchburg clearly were not the norm, it is important to understand the sources of such anomalies.

Having just highlighted the variation of experiences across cities, I would like now to return to the more general and surprising patterns shown in figures 1.1–1.3. The rapid improvements in urban black life expectancies shown in these figures are particularly surprising when one considers how historians typically portray black access to public health facilities, such as public water and sewer services. Consider, for example, the following summary of the historical literature on race, disease, and the provision of public health in American cities:

By the early 1900s, large American cities were so sharply segregated by class and race that the discrepancies between neighborhoods in both mortality rates and sanitary conditions were stark and alarming. Although reformers agitated to extend to poor neighborhoods municipal boons such as filtered water, adequate sewer connections, and garbage collection, the process was slow, largely because poor residents paid fewer taxes and had less political clout than did their affluent counterparts.[5]

Similarly, one urban historian suggests that black neighborhoods in Atlanta, Georgia, may have never received water and sewer service.[6] Along the same lines, a recent study of public health in Richmond, Virginia, finds that owing to "racial discrimination inherent in the system of healthcare delivery," the city's African-American community benefitted "only marginally" from the improvements in public health, including efforts to battle waterborne diseases such as typhoid fever.[7]

A few writers present slightly more optimistic pictures, showing that blacks received water, sewers, and other public health measures, but only when whites were able to internalize some benefits from extending these services to black communities. Usually these benefits stemmed from the reduced risk of epidemic diseases spreading from black neighborhoods to white ones.[8]

The idea that blacks had limited access to public water and sewer lines is not limited to urban and medical historians. In *Competition and Coercion*, Robert Higgs was the first historical economist to observe that there were dramatic reductions in black mortality during the late nineteenth and early twentieth centuries: "A variety of evidence points toward a significant reduction in black mortality during the period 1865–1914. The obvious question is: What accounts for this reduction?" Attributing the reduction in mortality to improved economic conditions among African Americans, Higgs explicitly rejects the idea that public health interventions played even a minor role in promoting black longevity. He characterizes public health interventions as unimportant because such "improvements made virtually no impact on the countryside before 1915," while "in the cities most blacks lived in slums or outlying areas poorly served by the new practices in sewerage and water supply."[9]

1.2 Solving the Puzzle of African-American Mortality

The simplest way to resolve the conflict between the data on life expectancy and the generally accepted historical observations is to challenge the data. This approach is unsatisfactory on at least three levels, however. First, the data that I use are the product of years of demographic research and by nearly all accounts provide a reasonably accurate measure of trends in life expectancy. Second, the patterns described here can be observed in a wide variety of data sources. As tables 1.1 and 1.2 suggest, these patterns can be observed in data aggregated at the federal, state, or local level; and they can be observed in the North and the South and in large and small cities. Because the patterns are so widespread and can be found in so many independent sources, it seems unlikely that they could be a statistical artifact or systematically biased in one direction or another.

Third, for years historians have been using the identical data to make the point that state and local officials discriminated in the provision of public health services. Historians often argue that interracial disparities in disease rates reflected inequities in the provision of such services. For example, between 1900 and 1920, blacks died of typhoid fever at roughly twice the rate that whites did.[10] Because typhoid was usually transmitted through water tainted by sewage, historians have attributed such differences to the failure of cities to install water and sewer mains in black neighborhoods.[11] The data that underlie this and other comparisons of black and white mortality are ultimately derived from the same sources as the data presented in this book. So if the data used here are flawed, the data that have allowed previous historians to routinely attribute interracial differences in disease rates to inequities in public services are also flawed. Setting aside genuine scientific concerns about data quality, this line of thought makes it impossible to say anything at all about the sources of interracial disparities in health.

Instead, I propose taking another look at the arguments historians have come to accept as fact. To be clear, this is not a proposal for wholesale revisionism and abandoning all that we currently know about African-American history. It is rather a proposal to reconsider a fairly modest and narrow set of facts: those associated with the provision of public water and sewer lines. Access to public water and sewer facilities was of central importance to the mortality of blacks and whites in turn-of-the-century America. In 1900, two waterborne diseases—typhoid and diarrhea—had a combined death rate of 186 deaths per 100,000 persons; only respiratory diseases such as tuberculosis and pneumonia killed more people. Moreover, waterborne disease rates alone understate the importance of water and sewer systems for morbidity and mortality, because as explained in chapter 2, even individuals who survived their bouts with typhoid and diarrhea in the short run had an elevated risk of heart disease later in life and would often later contract virulent cases of tuberculosis, pneumonia, or flu because their immune systems had been so compromised in fighting off typhoid.

The revisions I propose are as follows. During the late nineteenth and early twentieth centuries, racial inequities in the provision of public water and sewer facilities were much less pronounced than in other arenas, such as education and criminal justice. Indeed, in terms of disease reduction, African Americans benefitted more than whites when municipalities improved public water and sewer systems. Why did these systems differ so much from other public services? Public water and sewer systems were an exceptional case because discrimination in this arena was costly to white politicians and voters in at least three ways. First, given the networked structure of these systems, it was difficult to deny service to African-American households and neighborhoods without also denying service to white households and neighborhoods. This was particularly true during the late nineteenth century, when cities were much less segregated than they are today and when they were in the process of installing and extending water and sewer systems. Second, in a world where blacks and whites lived in close proximity, "sewers for everyone" was an aesthetically sound strategy. Third, failing to install water and sewer mains in black neighborhoods increased the risk of diseases spreading from black neighborhoods to white ones.

Collectively, these propositions help resolve the puzzling history of African-American longevity and suggest the following argument: The rapid *absolute* and *relative* improvements in health and life expectancy that occurred during the early twentieth century were driven in large part by the installation of water and sewer systems; by the 1960s, water and sewer systems were largely complete, and as a result the improvements in health slowed. It is important to emphasize that this argument applies only to African Americans living in urban areas. It cannot explain (the relatively limited) improvements in life expectancy that occurred among African Americans living in rural areas for the simple reason that water and sewer systems were not being built in unincorporated rural areas, for either whites or blacks. In 1920 about one-third of the African-American population lived in urban areas, and by 1940 about 48 percent lived in urban areas. Over the same 20-year period, the proportion of the white population living in urban areas remained constant, at roughly 55 percent.[12]

The argument that the absolute and relative improvements in black life expectancy were driven by the introduction of water and sewer service depends on two strong but I think legitimate propositions. The first is that water and sewer systems had large effects on human mortality and morbidity, regardless of race. In this regard, the estimates in chapter 3 suggest that about one-quarter of the decline in human mortality that occurred between 1900 and 1940 can be attributed to the elimination of diseases that are directly waterborne. However, this statistic alone understates the benefits of water and sewer systems. As shown in chapters 2 and 3, access to clean water promoted better overall health, less stress, and a bolstered ability to fight off other diseases, and in this way clean water reduced mortality from diseases that were not directly waterborne, such as heart disease and pneumonia. When one considers these secondary effects, the benefits of eliminating waterborne diseases were even larger. These statistics give force to the statements of Dr. Halden Mahler, the former director general of the World Health Organization, who has said that "the number of water taps per 1,000 persons is a better indicator of [a nation's] health than the number of hospital beds."[13]

The second critical proposition is that urban-dwelling blacks benefitted disproportionately from improvements in water and sewer systems. In this regard, chapter 6 shows that in the typical American city the installation of a water filter reduced the black death rate from typhoid by 53 percent, while it reduced white rates by only 16 percent. In some cities evidence of disproportionate benefits is even stronger. African Americans benefitted disproportionately from such investments because they were less able than whites, who were better informed and wealthier, to perform the household-level tasks needed to prevent typhoid, such as boiling water and purchasing bottled water. The idea that the household ability to prevent typhoid varied across socioeconomic groups is developed in chapter 3.

While these arguments challenge some generally accepted historical truths, they are not entirely new either. The arguments regarding the construction and extensiveness of urban water and sewer systems are reminiscent of Jon C. Teaford's claims in *The Unheralded Triumph: City Government in America, 1870–1900*. The arguments on the significance of disease spillovers complement a widely cited article by Stuart Galishoff, "Germs Know No Color Line: Black Health and Public Policy in Atlanta, 1900–1918" and a recent book by Don H. Doyle, *New Men, New Cities, New South*. The arguments regarding the efficacy of water purification, and the political and social determinants of infrastructure building, owe much to the work of Joel Tarr. The idea that blacks, as well as poor whites, were less able to engage in the household-level activities necessary to stave off typhoid fever has been explored in previous work by urban historians such as Clayton R. Koppes and William P. Norris and by historical demographers such as Samuel Preston, Michael Haines, Gretchen Condran, and Douglas Ewbank. Also, implicit throughout this book is the idea that people in cities in turn-of-the-century America were interconnected not just by germs, but by infrastructure, work, and geographic proximity. This line of thought parallels a central theme in *The Sanitary City* by Martin V. Melosi and in several other recent books on urban and technological history.

Finally, in his landmark book, *The Modern Rise of Population*, Thomas McKeown has shown that large reductions in human mortality occurred before the introduction of antibiotics, widespread immunizations, and effective clinical treatments of most diseases. Because these mortality reductions preceded effective medical therapies, McKeown argues that they must have been driven by environmental changes, particularly improved nutrition brought about partly by economic growth and the associated increases in food supplies, and to a lesser extent by improved public-health infrastructures such as public water and sewer lines. It is not possible to review all of the literature that has been generated by McKeown's work, but two articles by Simon Szreter are particularly relevant for the topics considered here. Szreter argues that McKeown simultaneously overstates the importance of economic growth and development in promoting health and understates the role of government investments in public infrastructure, especially water and sewer facilities.[14] The evidence presented here is consistent with the second part of Szreter's argument that public investments played a key role in reducing mortality and promoting longer life, especially for disadvantaged socioeconomic groups.[15]

1.3   The Contributions of This Book

With so many intellectual antecedents, one is tempted to ask what exactly is new here. What is new here is the basic thesis that African-American households in urban areas had greater access to public water and sewer systems than commonly believed, and that they actually benefitted disproportionately from such investments. To my knowledge, no previous historical work has stated, tested, and explored the generality of this hypothesis across cities and regions, or used such a wide variety of evidentiary sources as this book does. Along these lines, one of the questions raised by existing research centers around variation in the extensiveness and equity of water and sewer systems across cities. Put more simply, why did some cities, such as Memphis, Tennessee, build large and relatively equitable systems, while other cities, such as Savannah, Georgia, built less extensive and less equitable systems? The arguments developed here explain the intercity variation we observe in water and sewer systems. In particular, this book suggests that intercity differences in the level of residential segregation and in the magnitude of disease spillovers were important determi-

nants of the extensiveness and distributional fairness of urban water
and sewer systems. Understanding these forces can in turn help explain some of the intercity variation in the mortality of blacks highlighted in table 1.2 and discussed earlier.

More generally, the statistical and economic evidence offered later in
the book is particularly important. While statistical and econometric
methods play a vital and expanding role among demographers, economists, legal scholars, political scientists, and the like, historians have
largely abandoned numbers. This is unfortunate, because there are
many important historical questions for which there can be no substi-
tute for a quantitative approach. Such is the case here. Consider the oft-
repeated claim that "germs knew no color line." There is no question
that white public officials frequently said that diseases like tuberculosis
and cholera originated in black or poor immigrant neighborhoods and
subsequently spread to white.[16] However, in the absence of hard statistical evidence, it is impossible to know whether such statements
reflected fact, xenophobia, political opportunism, or some combination
of all three. And even if we could know, quotations are of little use in
assessing magnitudes. How extensive were disease spillovers? How
much lower would white disease rates have been if diseases had not
spread from black to white communities, and vice versa? How important were disease spillovers? Did they prompt local politicians to
spend public dollars in ways they otherwise would not have? The
answers to these questions are essential if we are to understand how
and why African-American life expectancy rose so sharply during the
early twentieth century, and yet these questions will remain unan-
swered if we rely exclusively on quotations and literary allusions.

1.4 Organization

The rest of the book proceeds as follows. Chapter 2 describes the epidemiology of diarrhea and typhoid fever. Particular attention is given
to the long-term health effects of these diseases, and the role public
water and sewer systems played in their eradication.

Chapter 3 describes the evolution of residential segregation, and the
concurrent development of water and sewer systems in major American cities. The chapter argues that public water and sewer systems
were built in an era of relatively low residential segregation, and that
this made it difficult to deny African-American neighborhoods access

to public water and sewer lines. Furthermore, access to public water and sewer services was especially beneficial for poor socioeconomic groups, like African Americans.

Chapter 4 presents case studies of Memphis, Tennessee; Savannah, Georgia; and Jacksonville, Florida. Memphis, the site of the worst epidemic in American history, caused by yellow fever, offers a natural place in which to explore the role that epidemic diseases played in motivating city officials to bring water and sewer service to African-American neighborhoods. Savannah, which also has a remarkable disease history, was more segregated than Memphis and helps identify the effects of segregation and disease spillovers in determining the choices of local water and sewer officials. The role that racism played in motivating public officials to extend water and sewer lines is explored through the case study of Jacksonville, and its municipal health officer, Dr. C. E. Terry, a dyed-in-the-wool racist.

Chapter 5 builds on the following logic: if discrimination was as severe in the provision of public water and sewer services as it was in education, there would have been as much litigation surrounding these facilities as there was surrounding education. A focal point of chapter 5 is the experience of Shaw, Mississippi, one of the few towns that have been found guilty of discriminating against black neighborhoods when it installed water and sewer mains. The case study of Shaw is buttressed by an econometric analysis of some 250,000 households.

The keystone of the book is chapter 6, where I analyze how variation in water quality affected racial disparities in waterborne disease rates. The econometric work explores how the introduction of public water filtration affected black and white typhoid rates in a panel of thirty-three American cities. If cities systematically denied African Americans access to public water systems, improvements in water quality (measured by the installation of a water filter) would have benefitted whites disproportionately. The econometric work in this chapter also identifies the size of disease spillovers, and the importance of residential segregation in protecting white communities against typhoid epidemics in black communities.

Because the statistical findings in chapter 6 are critical to my argument, I subject them to thorough scrutiny in chapter 7. In particular, chapter 7 considers three related issues: whether the statistical findings in chapter 6 withstand reasonable changes in the specification of my statistical model; whether the assumptions that motivate the empirical work in chapter 6 are reasonable; and whether the data employed in chapter 6 are reliable.

Chapter 8 uses cross-sectional data to explore how extensions in water systems affected black and white waterborne disease rates using cross-sectional data. In particular, it sets out to answer the question: did extensions in public water systems affect black waterborne disease rates disproportionately? It also considers the relationship between population growth and extensions in water systems. Suppose that when cities installed water mains, they focused only on demand for water in white neighborhoods and ignored demand in black neighborhoods. If so, growth in mains would have been much more responsive to changes in the white population than to changes in the black population.

Chapter 9 summarizes my findings.

2

Waterborne Diseases

2.1 Introduction

Much of my analysis focuses on disease rates, particularly those for waterborne diseases. A working knowledge of the epidemiology of such diseases is therefore essential. Accordingly, this chapter examines the two waterborne diseases that posed the greatest threat to the American population during the late nineteenth and early twentieth centuries: typhoid fever and diarrhea.[1] Because fecal contamination of food and water was the primary mode of transmission, public investments in water filtration and public sewer lines significantly reduced death rates from these diseases. Medical interventions did not play an important role in combating waterborne diseases during the early twentieth century.[2] An important subtheme of this chapter is that even if an individual survived bouts of typhoid fever and diarrhea in the short run, these illnesses often had severe long-term consequences. For example, typhoid fever adversely affected the long-term viability of several bodily functions and left survivors vulnerable to other diseases.

2.2 Typhoid Fever: Epidemiology, Symptoms, and Long-Term Effects

Epidemiology

During the late nineteenth and early twentieth centuries, the waterborne disease that posed the most serious threat to adult populations in America was typhoid fever. Typhoid fever is caused by *Salmonella typhi*, a bacterium that can survive only in human hosts and lives in the intestinal tract. People typically contracted the disease by drinking contaminated water. A common transmission might have gone like this: The family of a typhoid victim dumped the patient's waste into a cesspool or privy vault. If the vault was too shallow or had leaks, it seeped into underground water sources. If these water sources were not adequately filtered, people who drew their water from them contracted typhoid fever. A related mode of transmission occurred when surface privies were not screened. With open privies, flies would come in contact with the pathogens in human wastes and then transfer the germs to the kitchens of neighboring homes. Fly-transmitted infections appear to have been most common in the South, where the climate is conducive to the proliferation of insects.[3]

Although tainted drinking water and unsanitary disposal of sewage were the most frequent modes of transmission in the United States, typhoid spread through other means as well. Shellfish from tainted rivers and lakes carried typhoid. If they were washed or sprinkled with tainted water, raw fruits and vegetables carried the typhoid bacillus. Milk became a carrier when it was put in containers cleaned with tainted water or when the individuals who milked the cow did not adequately wash before milking. Typhoid was also spread through incidental, secondhand contact. Doctors, nurses, laundry workers—anyone who came in contact with the wastes of an infected person—could carry typhoid bacilli on their hands and clothes. Caregivers sometimes unwittingly transferred those germs to the eating utensils in their own homes, infecting themselves and other family members.[4]

In addition, in some cases people did not know they were infected with typhoid because the symptoms were so mild. These were called walking cases because the victims could continue to work and socialize. Walking cases occurred most frequently in children. In other cases, people harbored the typhoid bacillus without ever developing the disease. These people were called carriers. The phrase "typhoid Mary" originated with Mary Mallon, the first identified typhoid carrier in the United States. Although Mallon knew that she carried typhoid, she refused to stop working as a cook and reportedly infected more than fifty people during her life.[5]

During the late nineteenth and early twentieth centuries, typhoid was rarely diagnosed in children under the age of five, not because it never occurred in young children, but because it was very difficult to diagnose in the young. Finally, there are no known genetic or biological characteristics that leave one race or sex more susceptible to typhoid than another.[6]

The spread of typhoid is influenced by environmental and demographic factors. The disease thrives in warm climates, and in endemic areas peaks during the summer months. It is not clear what drives the correlation between temperature and typhoid. Warm temperatures might lead people to consume more water, increasing the likelihood that they will ingest the typhoid bacillus; or alternatively, warm temperatures encourage typhoid bacilli to proliferate in food and water. Typhoid also appears to be positively correlated with migration. Migrant populations are more susceptible to typhoid than are the native-born, who have developed resistance to the disease over time. While exposure to typhoid confers some immunity against future infection, this immunity declines over time and can be overcome at any point through exposure to a sufficiently large number of typhoid bacteria.[7]

To the extent that poverty is correlated with poor sanitation and health practices, typhoid is also positively correlated with poverty. This is evidenced by international comparisons of typhoid rates today. In well-developed areas, such as the United States, Europe, and Japan, the annual death rate from typhoid is less than 1 per 100,000 persons, while in lesser-developed areas, such as Africa and Southeast Asia, annual death rates range from 500 to 1,000 deaths per 100,000 persons.

Diagnosing Typhoid: A Description of Symptoms

Once they enter the body, typhoid bacilli have a 1- to 3-week incubation period. During incubation, an infected individual experiences mild fatigue, loss of appetite, and minor muscle aches. After incubation, the victim experiences more severe symptoms: chills, coated tongue, nosebleeds, coughing, insomnia, nausea, and diarrhea. At its early stages, typhoid's symptoms often resemble those of respiratory diseases, and pneumonia is often present. In nearly all cases, typhoid victims experience severe fever. Body temperatures can reach as high as 105°F. A week or so after incubation, rose-colored spots sometimes appear on the patient's abdomen. For much of the nineteenth century, these rose-colored rashes were the only symptom doctors could use to identify typhoid definitively, but unfortunately in terms of promoting accurate diagnoses, these rashes appear in only 5 to 20 percent of all cases.[8]

Three weeks after incubation, the disease is at its worst. The patient is delirious, emaciated, and often has blood-tinged stools. One in five typhoid victims experiences a gastrointestinal hemorrhage. Internal hemorrhaging results when typhoid bacilli perforate the intestinal wall and frequently continue on to attack the kidneys and liver. The risk of pulmonary complications, such as pneumonia and tuberculosis, is high at this time. Perhaps as many as two-thirds of the deaths associated with typhoid fever (in the turn-of-the-century United States) were not due directly to the effects of typhoid, but to tuberculosis, pneumonia, and other complications such as kidney and liver damage. The high fever associated with typhoid is so severe that about half of all victims experience neuropsychiatric disorders at the peak of the disease. These include encephalopathy (swelling of the brain), nervous tremors and other Parkinsonlike symptoms, abnormal behavior, babbling speech, confusion, and visual hallucinations. If, however, the patient survives all of this, the fever begins to fall off and a long period of recovery sets in. It can take as long as 4 months to fully recover. Surprisingly, given the severity of typhoid's symptoms, more than 90 percent of its victims during the nineteenth and twentieth centuries survived. But as explained later, this low case fatality rate understates the devastating effects of typhoid on a person's long-term health.[9]

Surviving Typhoid: Long-Term Effects

The fact that typhoid kills only 5 to 10 percent of its victims might lead one to wonder just how significant this disease could have been for human health and longevity in turn-of-the-century America. However, when typhoid does not kill its victims quickly and directly, it kills them slowly and indirectly, in a way that made it impossible for nineteenth-century observers to identify the real culprit. Accordingly, in this subsection I discuss the long-term health effects of exposure to typhoid. This discussion shows that exposure to typhoid and diarrhea at early stages in life increases the risk of heart disease, respiratory problems, neurological problems, and liver and kidney troubles in later years. If one considers the severity of typhoid's symptoms, which range from hallucinations to acute renal failure, it is not surprising that exposure to typhoid undermines a person's long-term health prospects.

Typhoid affects nearly all bodily systems and leaves many of them permanently damaged. The discussion here focuses on the cardiovascular, respiratory, gastroenterological, and neurological systems. In the case of the cardiovascular system, S. N. Khosla reports that 12 percent of typhoid patients studied during the mid-twentieth century experienced some sort of cardiac event while fighting off the disease.[10] Similarly, using a sample of records for nearly 30,000 Union Army recruits, Dora L. Costa shows that holding everything else constant, those who fell victim to typhoid during the Civil War had elevated rates of heart disease and heart trouble later in life. In particular, recruits who had typhoid fever had about a 25 percent higher risk of heart trouble later in life than those who had not experienced typhoid.[11]

As for typhoid's impact on respiratory function, probably the country's foremost expert on typhoid at the turn of the century, George C. Whipple, wrote: "It is said that not over a third of the deaths from typhoid fever are due directly to the effects of the disease, i.e., to the effects of the typho-toxin. Two-thirds of the deaths are due to the numerous complications, among which tuberculosis and pneumonia are prominent."[12] Elsewhere, Whipple explained that the risk of contracting pulmonary complications such as tuberculosis and pneumonia was especially high when typhoid was at its peak, around the second or third week of the illness.[13] With quotations it is always difficult to disentangle hyperbole from fact and so, based on Whipple's statement alone, one might be hesitant to push the case that surviving typhoid left one vulnerable to life-threatening attacks from pneumonia and tuberculosis. However, the general claim that typhoid adversely affected respiratory function receives support from Costa. Costa shows that wartime exposure to typhoid increased the risk of respiratory problems later in life by more than 50 percent.[14]

The fact that typhoid fever left the patient vulnerable to tuberculosis is doubly important because exposure to tuberculosis was like exposure to typhoid. If it did not kill you the first time, it killed you the second time. Again, Costa's study of the wartime disease experience of Union Army recruits is instructive. She found that recruits who contracted tuberculosis during the Civil War were about 25 percent more likely to have had an irregular pulse later in life and were twice as likely to have had decreased respiratory function later in life.[15] Costa's findings are supported by studies employing more modern data, which find a strong correlation between respiratory diseases in childhood and poor health later in life.[16]

In a recent paper with the apt title, "The Liver in Typhoid Fever: Always Affected, Not Just a Complication," R. Morgenstern and P. C. Hayes review the evidence documenting typhoid's effect on the liver. According to these authors, 90 percent of all typhoid cases had some degree of liver involvement, ranging from biochemical abnormalities to overt hepatitis; about 5 percent of all typhoid victims developed hepatitis.[17] Kidney problems were also common, ranging from swelling and high protein levels in the urine to full-blown nephritis. Studies of current populations suggest that at least 10 to 15 percent of typhoid victims would have experienced a significant abnormality in kidney function.[18] In one study performed during the 1990s, 79 percent of all typhoid victims exhibited symptoms consistent with urinary tract infections.[19] Today, complications with the kidney and liver can be managed through dialysis and drug treatment, limiting the long-term damage to these vital organs. However, among earlier populations, typhoid was allowed to run its course, and it seems likely that the disease would have left the kidneys and liver irreparably compromised in a large portion of the population that survived the short-term effects of the disease.

Studies of modern-day populations suggest that between 35 and 85 percent of all typhoid victims would have experienced some sort of neurological complications. These would have included severe confusion (30 to 70 percent of all cases), some type of swelling or inflamation of the brain or spinal chord (5 to 10 percent of all cases), and acute schizophrenia or psychosis (1 to 2 percent of all cases). Autopsies of people who have been killed by typhoid reveal diffuse damage to neurons, softening of the brain's vascular system, the formation of abscesses on the brain, and discharges of pus in the brain and meninges. For those who survived typhoid, all of these complications left scars and lesions.[20]

2.3   The Germ Theory of Disease and the Clinical Treatment of Typhoid

For much of the nineteenth century, people believed typhoid arose spontaneously or spread through miasmas—poisonous gases thought to rise from swamps, decaying matter, and filth. In 1840, William Budd challenged these ideas, showing that typhoid spread through water and food. Budd, an Englishman, recommended that the European governments invest in public health infrastructure to halt the spread of typhoid. However, scientists who continued to espouse the idea that typhoid arose spontaneously, or spread through miasmas, vigorously attacked Budd and his new theory. Because of their attacks, Budd's recommendations were not soon implemented, and typhoid rates in Europe remained as high as 500 deaths per 100,000 persons. It took more than three decades for Budd's theories and recommendations to take hold in England. In 1875, the British government finally passed the Public Health Act and began improving its public health systems. Ten years later, typhoid rates in England had fallen 50 percent.[21]

In the United States, the rise of the germ theory of disease in general, and Budd's ideas in particular, made it possible for doctors to better diagnose and treat typhoid. This pattern can be illustrated by exploring the problems doctors had in distinguishing between typhoid and malaria. For much of the nineteenth century, doctors often lumped together deaths associated with high fevers and diarrhea into one category referred to as "typhomalarial fever." The discoveries of scientists like Budd made it clear that while diseases like typhoid and malaria shared certain symptoms, they were in fact distinct diseases caused by two entirely different pathogens. They were not spread by the same mysterious poison floating in the air. Moreover, over the course of the late nineteenth century, doctors were able to distinguish typhoid from malaria in at least some cases because of the distinctive abdominal rash that sometimes developed in typhoid. By the turn of the twentieth century, doctors were able, at least in theory, to positively identify typhoid through the Widal test, a laboratory analysis of the blood or stools of ill patients. Such diagnostic tools were predicated on the understanding that typhoid was caused by a unique bacterium.[22]

It is important to point out, however, that mistakes in diagnosing typhoid persisted into the early twentieth century. As explained fully in chapter 7, during the early 1900s, most deaths attributed to malaria probably should have been attributed to typhoid fever. Mistaken diagnoses occurred when blood tests were not available, perhaps because the patient had already perished. In these situations, doctors had to rely on more primitive and less accurate diagnostic techniques. Mistaking typhoid for malaria was far more common in the South than in North because of the relatively high incidence of malaria in the former. In Mississippi, for example, malaria was the third leading cause of death in 1900.[23] Also, white public health officials claimed that black doctors were poorly trained and therefore diagnosed typhoid as malaria more frequently than white doctors. While these claims were largely the result of racist stereotypes and prejudices, it probably was the case that African Americans were more likely to have had their illnesses misdiagnosed because they were getting relatively low-quality care from physicians, if they were getting any care at all.[24] For example, evidence presented in chapter 7 shows that blacks were 3.5 times more likely than whites to have died without an attending physician.

Effective clinical treatments did not come on the scene until fairly late. Not until 1948, when doctors started giving typhoid victims the antibiotic chloramphenicol, did the medical community develop effective treatments for typhoid fever. If they were administered early in the onset of disease, antibiotics had a dramatic effect. They cut the case mortality rate to less than 1 percent and eliminated the fever within a few days. At the turn of the century, though, doctors could do little to help typhoid victims other than recommend bed rest and a healthy diet. As stated earlier, treated this way, typhoid killed 5 to 10 percent of its victims.[25]

Almroth Wright developed the first effective typhoid vaccine around 1900. Wright killed typhoid bacteria with heat and then used the dead bacteria to immunize patients. The vaccine had a protective effect of about 75 percent. While the vaccine could be produced cheaply and easily, it was costly to store and administer. It was given through three shots with a hypodermic needle, each shot 10 days apart. The vaccine also frequently caused adverse reactions, including high fever, soreness, nausea, vomiting, and headaches. In part because of these reactions and the vaccine's limited effectiveness, the Secretary of the Connecticut State Board of Health argued in 1913 that:

> It is not to be expected ... that typhoid vaccination will ever be used as is smallpox vaccination and depended upon for the eradication of typhoid, nor should it be. For that purpose we continue to depend on, and strive for, pure water, pure food, proper sewerage disposal, and other hygienic measures.[26]

Developed in England, the Wright vaccine did not gain popularity in the United States until World War I, when the American high command ordered mandatory vaccination for all soldiers.[27]

2.4 Preventing Typhoid

As the preceding discussion suggests, the most effective means of preventing typhoid was through improving local water systems, and there were two ways to do this. The first was through the extension of public water and sewer lines, which in urban areas gradually displaced the use of private surface wells and privy vaults. Water from private wells was rarely filtered and was not regularly tested for impurities, as was more often the case with water supplied by large water companies, whether public or private. The second, and related, way to improve local water supplies was to install filters and to chlorinate the water.

Extending Public Water Supplies

Writing at the turn of the twentieth century, state health departments suggested a causal link between access to public water systems and waterborne disease rates. Consider the following description of waterborne disease epidemics in Winston and Salem, two small towns in North Carolina: "In Winston and Salem not less than thirty sporadic cases have occurred during the past two years. All of these were in families using well water. In the houses of neighbors using water from the public supply not one case occurred."[28] Situations like this prompted officials to advocate the extension of public water systems and the abandonment of private wells: "We wish to put ourselves on record as favoring the use of public water supplies as against the water of wells. The water of the public supply may sometimes be dangerous, but that from [private] wells ... is much more apt to be so."[29] An official of the Massachusetts State Board of Health expressed the same argument:

the highest death rates in the state are ... in the towns that depend for water upon wells.... The town which had the highest death rate from typhoid fever ... was Ware, and in the fifteen years previous to 1886 the average number of deaths per 10,000 inhabitants was 16.5. In 1886 this town introduced a supply of water, and in the years since ... the number of deaths has fallen to 6.9, four-tenths as many as previously.[30]

The experience of New Orleans, Louisiana, further highlights the benefits of extending public water lines. Until around 1905, New Orleans had by far the least-developed water system of any large American city, with fewer than 150 miles of water mains. In 1907, for cities with populations greater than 300,000 persons, miles of water mains per 1,000 persons averaged 1.342, while New Orleans had only 0.502 mile of mains per 1,000 persons.[31] Before 1905, most residents of New Orleans used rainwater collected in cisterns, or well water, as their primary source of drinking water. But between 1905 and 1915, the size of the city's water system grew fourfold, a historically unprecedented increase. The rapid expansion in water mains was associated with sharp reductions in typhoid death rates. This can be seen in figure 2.1, which plots typhoid death rates in the city from 1890 through 1920. Notice that before the expansion of the water system beginning in 1905, typhoid death rates were rising steadily, from 20 per 100,000 persons to about 60 deaths per 100,000. This upward trend was reversed around

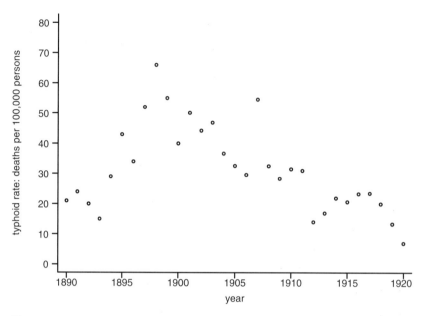

Figure 2.1
Typhoid fever in New Orleans, 1890–1920. Sources: Fuller, "Water-Works," p. 1220 and
U.S. Bureau of Census, *Mortality Statistics*, various years and *Census*, various years, vari-
ous volumes.

1905, when the rates began a steady and secular downward trend, falling to less than 10 deaths per 100,000 by 1920.[32]

Water Filtration

As stated earlier, the second way to eliminate typhoid was to install
water purification systems that used both filtration and chlorination.
The efficacy of these measures is illustrated in figures 2.2 and 2.3,
which plot typhoid death rates in Philadelphia, Pennsylvania, and
Chicago, Illinois, respectively. The vertical lines in both figures indicate
the installation of new water filters, the initiation of chemical steriliza-
tion, or changes to locate water intakes away from sewage-polluted
water sources. In Philadelphia, the installation of an extensive water
filtration system around 1908 was associated with a dramatic reduction in typhoid death rates. Before 1908, they never fell below 30
deaths per 100,000 persons, and were often between 60 and 80; after
1908, they never rose above 20 and began falling steadily. The introduction of chlorination in 1913 helped push typhoid death rates even

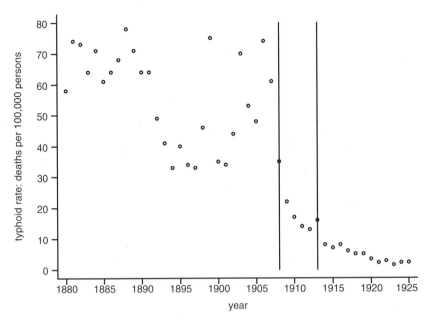

Figure 2.2
Typhoid fever and water filtration in Philadelphia, 1880–1925. The vertical lines indicate improvements in the city's water purification system. Sources: Fuller, "Water-Works," p. 1221; U.S. Bureau of Census, *General Statistics of Cities*, 1915 and *Mortality Statistics*, various years.

lower, and by 1920 the disease had been largely eradicated. Similarly, prior to the first improvement in the purity of Chicago's water in 1893, typhoid death rates in the city exhibited an upward trend, with the rates spiking to levels above 100 deaths per 100,000 persons in 3 years, and above 75 in 5 years. This upward trend was reversed in 1893 and after that year typhoid death rates never rose above 50 per 100,000 persons. Moreover, every subsequent improvement in the city's water purification system was associated with further reductions in typhoid, until 1920, when typhoid deaths in the city were effectively zero.[33] Additional and more powerful evidence of the effects of pure water on typhoid death rates is presented in chapter 6.

2.5 Diarrhea

The waterborne disease that killed the most people of any age in the late nineteenth and early twentieth centuries was diarrhea. However, diarrheal deaths occurred primarily among children less than 2 years

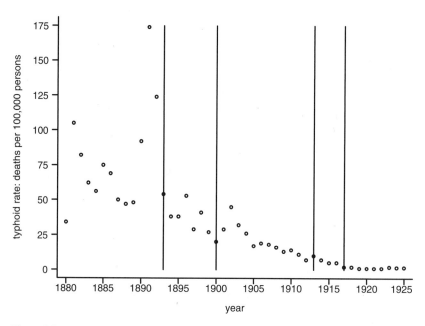

Figure 2.3
Typhoid fever and water filtration in Chicago, 1880–1925. The vertical lines indicate improvements in the city's water purification system. Sources: Fuller, "Water-Works," p. 1220; U.S. Bureau of Census, *General Statistics of Cities*, 1915 and *Mortality Statistics*, various years.

of age, and diarrheal illness was probably the leading cause of death for the very young. For example, a study of infant mortality in Baltimore, Maryland, conducted in 1915 found that 43 percent of all infant deaths were the result of diarrhea. Exactly how many of these deaths were the direct result of impure water is unclear. At the time, many public health experts believed that impure milk was a major cause of infantile diarrhea. The basis for this belief was that breast-fed infants had significantly lower mortality rates from diarrhea than infants fed with cow's milk.[34]

On the other hand, some of the infantile deaths attributed to diarrhea were almost certainly typhoid fever, but because of the difficulties of diagnosing typhoid at the time, particularly among the very young, these deaths were mistakenly attributed to diarrhea. As noted earlier, typhoid was never diagnosed in children less than five years old. Moreover, typhoid was sometimes transmitted through impure milk, and the correlation between breast-feeding and low infant mortality might partly reflect the fact that children were much more likely to

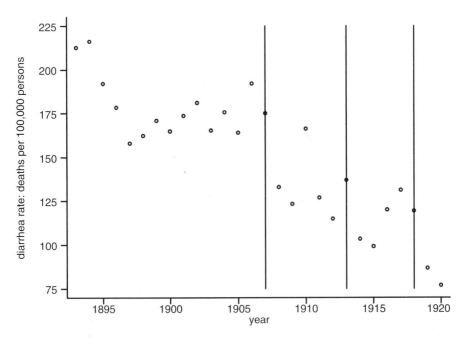

Figure 2.4
Diarrhea and water filtration in Pittsburgh, 1893–1920. The vertical lines indicate improvements in the city's water purification system. Sources: City of Pittsburgh, *Annual Report of the Department of Public Health* (various years); U.S. Bureau of Census, *General Statistics of Cities*, 1915 and *Mortality Statistics*, various years.

have been exposed to typhoid through cow's milk than through mother's milk. Finally, the correlation between breast-feeding and infant health is not limited to diarrhea. Infants who were breast-fed also had significantly lower nondiarrheal death rates than infants who were fed cow's milk.[35]

Given the questions raised about nonwater-related disease vectors in the case of diarrhea, it is useful to evaluate the relative importance of waterborne and nonwaterborne sources of diarrhea. I present four pieces of evidence on this issue. First, the econometric evidence presented in chapters 7 and 8 makes it clear that changes in water quality had a large and statistically significant effect on overall waterborne disease rates (i.e., typhoid and diarrhea). Second, figure 2.4 plots deaths from diarrhea in Pittsburgh, Pennsylvania, from 1893 through 1920. The figure also indicates the installation of new water filters and/or chlorination in Pittsburgh with three vertical lines. This figure suggests that deaths from diarrhea were highly correlated with water quality. Between 1893 and 1907, the diarrheal death rate never fell below 150 deaths per 100,000. After Pittsburgh installed its first water filter in 1908, the death rate fell about 20 percent. Further improvements in water quality in 1913 and 1918 reduced the death rate from diarrhea another 40 percent. Moreover, except for the 1890s,[36] it appears that the death rate from diarrhea would have shown little improvement without these improvements in water quality. Studies of Boston, Massachusetts, and Cincinnati, Ohio, also show that infant deaths were reduced following improvements in the public water and sewer systems.[37]

The third source of evidence is a brief review of the voluminous literature on the determinants of infant mortality. This literature suggests that among both modern-day and historical populations the introduction of public water and sewer lines has reduced infant deaths from diarrheal diseases, but that the efficacy of these interventions has varied across time and space. For example, studying a sample of nearly ten thousand women from urban Brazil during the 1970s, Thomas Merrick found that access to piped water explained about 20 percent of the variation in infant deaths. Merrick, however, found that familial characteristics such as maternal literacy had a larger effect than piped water.[38] Using household-level data from multiple countries in Africa, Asia, and the Americas during the 1980s, S. A. Esrey found that access to clean water and sanitary sewers resulted in significantly lower infant deaths and increased height and body weight for infants, adding perhaps as much as 1 to 2 kilograms to an infant's weight.[39] In a study of German cities between 1870 and 1910, John Brown found that about 40 percent of the reduction in childhood mortality that occurred over this period could be attributed to improvements in public water and sewer systems.[40]

To my mind, two of the best studies of the effects of access to public water supplies on infant mortality are of recent origin. In particular, Tara Watson examined how the introduction of piped water affected infant mortality rates on American Indian reservations during the 1970s. She finds that a 10 percent increase in the number of homes with improved public water and sewer access reduced infant mortality rates by about 4 percent. The second study is a jointly authored paper examining the effect of improvements in public water systems in Argentina. These improvements followed a wave of privatizations in the water industry during 1990s. The results of this study indicate that the improvements that stemmed from privatizing water systems reduced infant mortality rates by an average of 8 percent. The authors find, however, that the benefits of improved water systems were greatest for the poorest regions, which on average realized a 26 percent reduction in infant mortality.[41]

The fourth source of evidence is the study of infant mortality in Baltimore conducted by the Children's Bureau of the U.S. Department of Labor. This bureau performed a detailed censuslike study linking infant mortality with such factors as income, ethnicity, and public sewer connections. The study followed the birth and health of a large sample of infants born in Baltimore during 1915. Before presenting and describing the data from this study, a caveat needs to be noted. For reasons that are not clear, the bureau excluded from much of their published data infants who did not live more than 2 weeks. In the following analysis then, infants who died within the first 2 weeks of life are treated in the data as never having been born, and all results are subject to a concern about selection bias. Nonetheless, while the resulting measures cannot tell us about neonatal mortality, they do provide a reasonably good indicator of postneonatal infant mortality.[42]

The published data from the bureau's Baltimore study are only available in cells representing clusters of households with similar characteristics. There are fifty-one cells and these cells serve as the units of observation in the empirical work described here. Each cell is defined by its racial or ethnic characteristics, income, and connection to public sewers. There are six different racial or ethnic categories: black, native-born white, Italian immigrant, Jewish immigrant, Polish immigrant, and other immigrant.[43] There are seven income categories: less than $550 per year, between $550 and $849, between $850 and $1,249, between $1,249 and $1,849, more than $1,850, no income, and income not reported.[44] For example, the first cell reported by the Children's Bureau contains data on black households earning less than $550 a year, who were not connected to public sewers. Of the 581 infants born to Baltimore households with these characteristics in 1915, 11.5 percent died within the first year of life and 3.8 percent died of diarrhea. There is a great deal of variation in the number of births across cells, ranging from a low of 3 (multiple cells) to a high of 1,528.

With these data, variants on the following equation are estimated:

$$y = \beta_0 + \beta_1\chi_1 + \beta_2\chi_2 + \beta_3\chi_3 + \beta_4\chi_4 + \varepsilon, \tag{2.1}$$

where y is the postneonatal diarrheal infant mortality rate measured as the proportion of all live infants dying from diarrhea in the cell; χ_1 is a

Table 2.1
Infant Deaths from Diarrhea, and Access to Public Sewers in Baltimore

Variable	Unweighted regressions			Weighted regressions[a]		
	Mean (S.D.)	1a	1b	Mean (S.D.)	2a	2b
Diarrhea death rate[b]	0.040 (0.066)	Dependent variable		0.029 (0.025)	Dependent variable	
=1 if connected to public sewer	0.471 ...	−0.034* (0.015)	−0.030* (0.015)	0.434 ...	−0.017* (0.004)	−0.016* (0.004)
Nondiarrhea death rate[c]	0.058 (0.077)	...	0.140 (0.112)	0.038 (0.025)	...	0.044 (0.121)
Race dummies	...	Yes	Yes	...	Yes	Yes
Income dummies	...	Yes	Yes	...	Yes	Yes
Adjusted R^2	...	0.362	0.372	...	0.683	0.675
No. of observations	51	51	51	51	51	51

Source: See text.
Notes: An asterisk indicates significant at the 1 percent level or higher (one-tailed test). Standard deviations (S.D.) or standard errors are in parentheses.
[a] Regressions have been weighted by the number of births in each cell.
[b] Proportion of all infants living past 2 weeks who died from diarrhea during 1915.
[c] Proportion of all infants living past 2 weeks who died from nondiarrheal causes in 1915.
..., not applicable.

vector of dummy variables describing the race or ethnicity of the households in the cell; χ_2 is a vector of dummy variables indicating the income class of the cell; χ_3 is a dummy variable indicating access to sewers for households in the cell; χ_4 is the postneonatal nondiarrheal infant mortality rate measured as the proportion of all live infants dying from nondiarrheal diseases in the cell; and ε is a random-error term. The inclusion of the nondiarrheal death rate as an explanatory variable helps control for the general healthfulness of households contained in the cell. General healthfulness refers to a wide range of potential determinants of infant health, including feeding habits, genetic predispositions to premature death, sanitary characteristics of households, and the amount of crowding. Also, some regressions are weighted by the number of births in each cell. This controls for the fact that the true relationships among the variables will be measured with greater accuracy in cells for which there are large numbers of births.

If diarrhea shared the same basic epidemiology as typhoid, and was spread largely through fecal contamination, access to public sewers would have substantially reduced infant deaths from diarrhea. This suggests that the coefficient on the sewer dummy would be negative and large in terms of its absolute value. The dummy variables on ethnicity are important because the practice of breast-feeding varied across ethnic groups, and therefore these dummies capture and control for some of the effects of breast-feeding, along with the nondiarrheal death rate.[45]

The results are presented in table 2.1 and provide strong support for the idea that fecal matter was an important transmission mechanism for diarrheal diseases. In the unweighted regressions, the coefficient estimates suggest that sewer connections reduced the diarrheal death rate by 75 to 85 percent from its mean levels. Notice that adding the death rate from nondiarrheal causes, which is a crude way to control for unobserved differences in the level of healthfulness across populations, does not alter the conclusion that sewers mattered (see regressions 1a and 1b). In the weighted regressions, the estimates suggest that sewer connections reduced the diarrheal death rate by 55 percent from its mean level. Again, adding the death rate from nondiarrheal causes does not alter this conclusion.

2.6 Conclusions

This chapter shows that because typhoid fever and diarrhea were spread primarily through water tainted by human waste, or more generally, by human waste improperly disposed of, the construction of public water and sewer systems greatly reduced the death rate from these diseases. Examples from New Orleans, Chicago, and Philadelphia demonstrate the benefits of improving public water and sewer systems. Data from a study of infant mortality in Baltimore show how access to public water and sewer lines dramatically reduced infant deaths from diarrhea. This chapter also presents evidence that vaccinations and antibiotic medicines played a secondary role in eliminating typhoid fever. There was no vaccine for diarrhea, and the efficacy of antibiotic treatments for diarrhea depends on the extent to which the case in question is bacterial or viral. Moreover, an important subtheme of this chapter has been that typhoid has severe long-term consequences, even when it does not kill directly. Finally, this chapter shows that the ability to diagnose typhoid improved over time with the development of the germ theory of disease. The importance of this issue is discussed in chapter 7.

3

Sewers: When, Where, and to What Effect?

3.1 Introduction

This chapter explores the timing, location, and health effects of the construction of public water and sewer systems in American cities. After providing a brief overview of the history of residential segregation in America, the chapter presents evidence that in major American cities, public water and sewer systems were largely complete by around 1920, and that there was near racial parity in access to public water and sewer lines. The final sections explore the role that improvements in public water and sewer systems played in promoting American longevity between 1900 and 1940. Special attention is given to the experience of African Americans, and it is argued that the benefits of public water and sewer systems were particularly large for blacks and other disadvantaged groups, because socially constructed obstacles reduced the ability of the disadvantaged to prevent disease through private means.

3.2 Residential Segregation in America, 1890–2000

The idea that cities effectively denied African Americans access to water and sewer services assumes that cities were highly segregated and that the patterns of segregation were static. Because these services were distributed through a network of mains, it would have been difficult to discriminate against blacks without also adversely affecting whites if whites and blacks lived on the same streets and in close proximity to one another. Moreover, the patterns of segregation must have been static for the discrimination to have had permanent effects. If residential patterns evolved over time, so that white neighborhoods gradually became black neighborhoods, blacks would have acquired water and sewer services when they moved into better-served white neighborhoods.

Three Propositions about the History of Residential Segregation in America

It is difficult to generalize about the evolution of racial segregation in housing, but to the extent generalization is possible, three patterns appear to hold. First, cities were much less segregated during the nineteenth century than they are today. In 1890, the average black lived in a city ward that was only 20 percent black; by 1970, the average black lived in a ward that was 70 percent black.[1] More formal measures of housing segregation developed by historians and historical demographers, such as the index of dissimilarity and the index of isolation, yield the same conclusion.[2] (Because this generalization is central to my larger argument, it is explored in greater detail in the following section.) Second, segregation was more pronounced in the North and in large, fast-growing cities.[3] Third, after Reconstruction, black populations tended to concentrate on the periphery of southern cities and towns; only affluent whites could afford lots within walking distance of central business districts. Over the next hundred years, however, this pattern was reversed, as blacks moved into central cities and whites moved to suburbs.[4]

Although segregated housing patterns began to emerge soon after the Civil War, an important factor in the rise of segregation was the passage of "segregation laws" around 1910. At this time, cities throughout the South enacted municipal ordinances prohibiting individuals who lived on a street where the majority of homes were already owned by one race from selling their homes to another race (e.g., whites to blacks and vice versa).[5] While C. Vann Woodward has argued that local laws in the post-Reconstruction South often codified existing norms and customs, a recent econometric study suggests that segregation laws and other formal legal institutions were the driving force behind the emergence of segregated housing patterns during the early twentieth century.[6]

Further Thoughts on the Increasing Level of Residential Segregation in American Cities

The idea that cities became increasingly segregated over time is an essential part of the analysis that follows and requires additional elaboration and evidence. But first a caveat should be noted. The statement that cities became increasingly segregated over time should not be taken to imply that nineteenth-century cities in the American South were not segregated along racial lines, because they were. However, the type of segregation that existed in 1870 and 1880 was qualitatively different from that seen a century later. Racial segregation in the recent past can be observed at high levels of geographic aggregation such as entire city wards or census tracts. In contrast, during the nineteenth century, segregation was typically seen at much finer levels of aggregation so that parts of alleys, streets, or blocks were largely black or largely white.[7]

In major cities, there was no single area referred to as the African-American side of town. Instead, African-American neighborhoods were spread across town. For example, John Kellog explored the development of African-American neighborhoods in the following southern cities around 1900: Lexington, Kentucky; Atlanta, Georgia; Durham, North Carolina; and Richmond, Virginia. In Lexington, Kellog identified thirty-one separate African-American neighborhoods. These neighborhoods were distinct units and were spread evenly throughout Lexington and its periphery, although only two were near the city's central business district. In Atlanta, he identified twenty-four neighborhoods, again spread throughout the city and its periphery, except for the city's central business district. In Richmond, these patterns are repeated once again. As of 1900, there were thirty-two distinct African-American neighborhoods, and they were spread throughout the city except for the central business district. Only in Durham were the patterns different. In Durham, there were only eleven African-American neighborhoods and these were all located toward the center of town. The case studies of Memphis, Tennessee, and Savannah, Georgia, in chapter 4 corroborate the findings of Kellog and other historical geographers.[8]

3.3 Water and Sewer Systems in Turn-of-the-Century America

This section documents the extensiveness of urban water and sewer systems in turn-of-the-century America. What becomes clear from this documentation, when viewed in the light of our brief history of residential segregation, is that water and sewer systems in major American cities were built in an era of relatively little residential segregation and that most systems were built and nearly complete before cities started passing segregation ordinances in 1910. And as explained earlier, the fact that water and sewer mains were built during an era of relatively low residential segregation is significant in at least two ways. First, low levels of segregation facilitated the spread of diseases from black neighborhoods to white. Statistical evidence presented in chapter 6 corroborates this view. The rate at which typhoid fever spread from black households to white ones was significantly higher in integrated cities than in segregated ones. In the presence of disease spillovers, city authorities had strong incentives to extend water and sewer lines to black households.

Second, given the networked structure of water and sewer main systems, residential integration made it difficult to avoid installing mains in black neighborhoods without also adversely affecting service to white neighborhoods. This point is illustrated in chapter 4 in a discussion on George Waring, a sanitary engineer who designed sewer systems for several medium-sized American cities, including Memphis, Tennessee; Owensboro, Kentucky; and Norfolk, Virginia. Examining Waring's designs and reading the text accompanying them, it is clear that basic engineering concerns overrode all other considerations. For example, when Waring discussed where mains should be laid, he made no mention of the people who lived there, or their race. Instead, he focused on such things as terrain, soil quality, elevation, and the need to install pumps in some areas in order that the sewers might drain properly.[9]

Access to Public Water and Sewer Systems

To identify the extensiveness of sewer and water systems, data are taken from the *General Statistics of Cities*. Compiled by the U.S. Bureau of the Census in 1909 and again in 1915, this source is subject to two caveats. First, the *General Statistics of Cities* presents statistics on sewer and water systems only for cities with populations greater than 30,000. This is important because evidence presented later suggests that small municipalities had less extensive water and sewer systems than large cities. Second, the data on sewer and water systems contained in the *General Statistics of Cities* are not based on the detailed household-level surveys people typically equate with the Bureau of the Census. They are, instead, based on the estimates of the local officials who replied to the surveys and questionnaires submitted by the bureau. Having said this, the accuracy of the data contained in these volumes can be verified by comparing them with other independent sources and studies.

Table 3.1
Proportion of Households with Public Water and Sewer Connections, circa 1910

Proportion of households connected to	Percentile						
	5th	10th	25th	50th	75th	90th	95th
Public sewers in 1909							
Full sample ($N = 158$)	0.26	0.43	0.63	0.78	0.89	0.97	0.98
North ($N = 135$)	0.23	0.43	0.63	0.79	0.91	0.97	0.99
South ($N = 23$)	0.29	0.49	0.59	0.70	0.85	0.87	0.88
Public water in 1915							
Full sample ($N = 152$)	0.67	0.75	0.86	0.95	1.00	1.00	1.00
North ($N = 124$)	0.67	0.75	0.85	0.95	1.00	1.00	1.00
South ($N = 28$)	0.70	0.78	0.87	0.95	1.00	1.00	1.00

Source: U.S. Bureau of Census, *General Statistics of Cities*, 1909 and 1915 volumes. Data prepared by the Center for Population of Economics, University of Chicago.

As explained later, such comparisons indicate that while the data contained in the *General Statistics of Cities* are somewhat more pessimistic than other sources regarding access to public water and sewer facilities, they are accurate and reliable.

Table 3.1 presents data on access to public sewers in 1909 and access to public water in 1915. By 1909, 50 percent of American cities had more than 78 percent of their population connected to local sewer systems. Although connection rates were slightly lower in the South, southern cities were not underdeveloped in terms of their sewer systems compared with northern cities. This is notable given the typical perception of the South as an economic and political backwater. If historical trends in the growth of household connections to sewers are projected forward, the median city would have had 100 percent of its population connected by 1914. The same linear projections suggest that even cities in the bottom 5 percent of the rankings—i.e., those with less than 26 percent of their populations connected to public sewers in 1909—would have had 100 percent connection rates before 1940.

Similar patterns hold in the provision of water in cities with populations greater than 30,000. By 1915, 50 percent of American cities had at least 95 percent of their populations connected to public water supplies, and even cities at the bottom of the distribution had connection rates of nearly 70 percent. Again, the South and the North appear nearly identical in terms of the development of their infrastructures. These data make a simple but important point. In major U.S. cities by

1920, most urban households had been connected to public water and sewer systems.

Regarding public water systems, it is also useful to highlight the extent to which public water companies took steps to guarantee the purity of the water they distributed. As of 1915, 47 percent of all cities (with populations greater than 30,000) used filtration and/or chlorination to purify their water. But this statistic significantly understates access to pure water because most cities that did not filter or chlorinate their water used underground water sources (wells or springs) that were largely free from bacterial pollution. Considering this, 76 percent of all cities distributed pure water either because they treated it or because they drew their water from pollution-free underground sources.

The statistics presented here are similar but slightly less optimistic than those presented by Joel Tarr and Martin V. Melosi, the leading historians of urban water and sewer systems in America today. In *The Search for the Ultimate Sink*, Tarr estimates that in 1890, 22.5 million individuals in the United States were connected to public water lines, while at the same time reporting that the urban population was 22.1 million. Tarr's data for sewers suggest that in 1910 between 83 and 99 percent of the urban population was connected to sewer lines, and his data for 1920 suggest that 88 percent of the urban population was connected to sewers.[10] In *The Sanitary City*, Melosi presents data suggesting that by 1914, 41 percent of the urban population was supplied with filtered water. Melosi's data for sewers suggest that by 1920, 87 percent of the urban population was connected to sewers and that by 1940, 95 percent of the urban population was connected to sewers.[11]

City Size and Access to Public Water and Sewer Systems

The extensiveness of urban water and sewer systems varied positively with city size. Or more precisely, the probability of living in a city with an incomplete water or sewer system fell as city size grew. This can be seen in figures 3.1 and 3.2. Figure 3.1 plots the percentage of households connected to public sewers as of 1909 against city size.[12] Outliers—that is, cities with unusually small sewer systems given their size—are indicated by partial name. Other cities are represented by small circles. Ignoring the outliers for the moment, the combined data fall into a triangular shape, so that as city size increases, the probability of having only a small proportion of the population connected to sewer lines falls. To see this, note the following pattern: For cities between

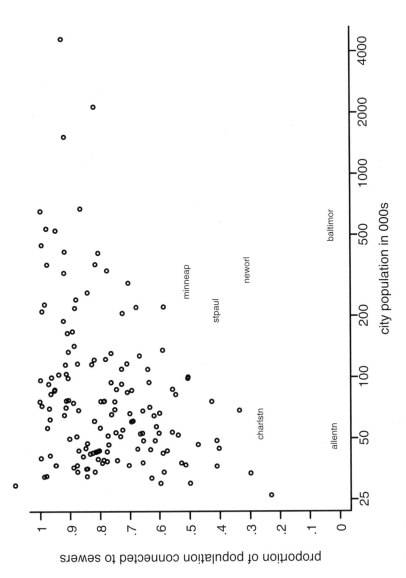

Figure 3.1
Access to public sewers in American cities, 1909. Cities with unusually incomplete systems indicated by partial name: Minneapolis, St. Paul, Charleston, New Orleans, Allentown, and Baltimore. The x-axis has a logarithmic scale. Source: U.S. Bureau of Census, *General Statistics of Cities*, 1909. Data prepared by Center for Population Economics, University of Chicago.

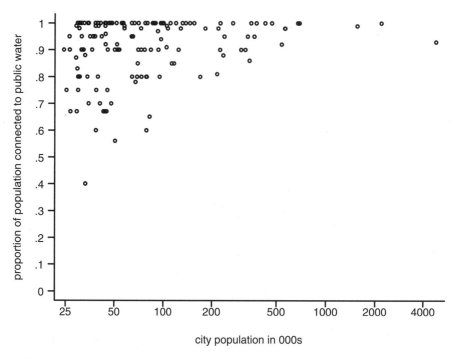

Figure 3.2
Access to public water supplies in American cities, 1915. The *x*-axis has a logarithmic scale. Source: U.S. Bureau of Census, *General Statistics of Cities*, 1915. Data prepared by Center for Population Economics, University of Chicago.

30,000 and 50,000 persons, the least-developed sewer systems extended to only 20 to 40 percent of the population; for cities between 100,000 and 200,000, the least-developed sewer systems extended to 50 to 60 percent of the population; for cities between 200,000 and 500,000, the least-developed sewer systems extended to 60 to 70 percent of the population; and for cities above 500,000, the least-developed sewer systems extended to no less than 80 percent of the population. Again, however, this discussion ignores outliers. These include Allentown, Pennsylvania; Baltimore, Maryland; Charleston, South Carolina; Minneapolis, Minnesota; New Orleans, Louisiana; and St. Paul, Minnesota. Notably, outliers are not limited to cities in the South.

Figure 3.2 plots the percentage of households connected to public water lines as of 1915 against city size. The same pattern emerges in the case of water as that for sewers. Again, the combined data fall into a triangular shape, so that as city size increases, the probability of having only a small proportion of the population connected to water lines falls. For cities between 30,000 and 50,000 persons, the least-developed water systems extended to 40 to 60 percent of the population; for cities between 100,000 and 200,000, the least-developed water systems extended to 60 to 80 percent of the population; for cities between 200,000 and 500,000, the least-developed water systems extended to 80 percent of the population; and for cities above 500,000, the least-developed water systems extended to no less than 90 percent of the population.

There are at least three possible explanations for the positive correlation between city size and the extensiveness of public water and sewer systems. First, it seems reasonable to assume that the risk of epidemic diseases varied positively with city size. That is, the risk of epidemics breaking out and spreading rapidly across the population was larger the larger and more densely populated the city. If this assumption is correct, and there is evidence to suggest that it is,[13] large cities would have had a stronger incentive to install extensive water and sewer systems, as well as other public health infrastructures, than did small cities. Second, given the large fixed costs associated with installing water and sewer systems, there were substantial economies of scale in the provision of these services. As a result, the per unit costs of providing water and sewer lines fell as population expanded, and it was more economical for large cities to install these systems than it was for small ones. Third, cities might have grown large because their governments offered various amenities. To the degree that the extensiveness of public water and sewer systems reflected the tendencies of local governments to offer such amenities, figures 3.1 and 3.2 might simply reflect the tendency of people to collect in attractive places. The problem with this line of thought is that places like New York and Philadelphia were large before they built their public infrastructures. Urban growth preceded urban infrastructure, not the other way round.[14]

3.4   Race and Access to Public Water and Sewer Lines: A Brief Introduction

In light of this book's focus on discrimination, it would be desirable to have information on the rates at which both black and white households were connected to public water and sewer lines. While such data are difficult to come by, some reliable sources of evidence are available. In chapter 4, I present detailed case studies of Memphis and Savannah, and for both of these cities I have precise information about access to water and sewer lines across racial groups. Here the focus is on two studies conducted by the Children's Bureau of the U.S. Department of Labor during the 1910s and 1920s, and on an investigation conducted jointly by the U.S. Department of Labor and Atlanta University in 1897. This study will be referred to as the Negro Mortality Project (NMP). The data from the latter are especially interesting because they provide evidence on numerous cities before the rapid expansion of the public water and sewer systems during the early 1900s.

In larger studies of the determinants of infant mortality, the Children's Bureau conducted detailed censuslike surveys of Baltimore, Maryland, in 1915 and Gary, Indiana, in 1922.[15] Through these surveys, the bureau gathered data on the rates at which black and white households in these cities were connected to local water and sewer systems. Gary and Baltimore are especially attractive for the purposes of this study because both cities ranked well below average in terms of the extensiveness of their water and sewer systems. In terms of the proportion of the local population connected to its sewer system, Baltimore ranked second to last of all large American cities; in 1909, less than 2 percent of Baltimore households were connected to public sewers. Only Allentown, Pennsylvania, had a less extensive sewer system. (The extent to which Baltimore lagged behind other cities in building sewers is demonstrated visually in figure 3.1.) Similarly, Gary was not incorporated until 1909 and did not begin building its water and sewer systems until that year.

Table 3.2 reports the results of the bureau's surveys. In Baltimore in 1915, 30 percent of black and 43 percent of white households were connected to public sewers. If historical trends continued, 100 percent of black households would have been connected to sewers by 1927, and 100 percent of white households by 1922. In Gary in 1922, 55 percent of black and 66 percent of white households were connected to sewers, while 69 percent of black and 75 percent of white households were connected to water mains. If historical trends continued, 100 percent of black households would have been connected to sewers by 1932, and 100 percent of white households by 1928. By 1929, 100 percent of black households would have been connected to public water mains, with 100 percent of white households connected by 1926. These linear projections in growth suggest that even in cities with very underdeveloped water and sewer systems (such as Baltimore and Gary), black households were connected to public water and sewer lines no more than 5 years after white households.

Table 3.2
Access to Public Water and Sewer in Baltimore and Gary, circa 1920

	Baltimore, 1915		Gary, 1922	
	Black	White	Black	White
Proportion of households				
Connected to public sewers	30%	43%	55%	66%
Connected to public water	n.a.	n.a.	69%	75%
Projected year when 100% of house-holds would have been connected to				
Public sewers	1927	1922	1932	1928
Public water	n.a.	n.a.	1929	1926

Sources: U.S. Department of Labor, Children's Bureau, *Results of a Field Study in Baltimore*, p. 213 and *Children of Preschool Age in Gary*, p. 62.
Note: n.a., not available.

Finally, consider the NMP's detailed study of African-American housing conditions in 1897.[16] Conducted under the auspices of prominent African-American leaders, the NMP was a detailed censuslike investigation of 1,137 black families. It surveyed families in seventeen southern cities and towns, and one northern city, Cambridge, Massachusetts. Census takers sometimes canvassed more than one neighborhood in each city. They also gathered household-level information about income, occupation, employment of spouse and children, health and sickness, and of particular importance, connections to public water and sewer lines. A more complete description and analysis of the NMP data is presented in the appendix.

Table 3.3 reports the results of the NMP survey regarding black access to public water and sewer systems in 1897. The survey indicates that even before the rapid expansion of public water and sewer systems during the early 1900s, a substantial fraction of all African-American families had access to public water and sewer lines. More precisely, the original NMP estimates suggest that in Cambridge and Washington, D.C., more than 90 percent of all households surveyed were connected to public water and sewer lines, although in the modal city, no households were connected. However, as explained in the appendix, these estimates probably understate access because of the surveying techniques employed by NMP investigators. These techniques involved surveying clusters of homes in particular neighborhoods, rather than broad cross sections of the local black population. Once one adjusts for this clustering, it appears that the typical city would have

Table 3.3
Connections to Public Water and Sewer Lines among Black Families in 1897

City	Total city population, 1890	Proportion of families with public water and sewer access			
		Original NMP estimate	"Declustered" estimates		
			1	2	3
Orangeburg, S.C.	2,964	0.000	0.000	0.000	0.000
Athens, Ga.	8,634	0.063	0.242	0.224	0.063
Cartersville, Ga.	3,171	0.000	0.350	0.326	0.185
Jacksonville, Fla.	17,201	0.359	0.359	0.335	0.196
Jackson, Tenn.	10,039	0.000	0.381	0.355	0.220
Atlanta, Ga.	65,514	0.128	0.491	0.460	0.346
Macon, Ga.	22,746	0.000	0.515	0.482	0.373
Nashville, Tenn.	76,168	0.004	0.555	0.519	0.419
Louisville, Ky.	161,129	0.000	0.591	0.552	0.459
Savannah, Ga.	43,174	0.012	0.805	0.754	0.703
Birmingham, Ala.	26,178	0.000	0.818	0.766	0.717
Cambridge, Mass.	70,082	0.979	0.979	0.917	0.900
Washington, D.C.	230,392	1.000	1.000	1.000	1.000
Chattanooga, Tenn.	29,100	0.000	n.a.	n.a.	n.a.
Columbia, S.C.	15,353	0.000	n.a.	n.a.	n.a.
Macon, Miss.	1,565	0.235	n.a.	n.a.	n.a.
Sanford, Fla.	2,016	0.125	n.a.	n.a.	n.a.
Tuskegee, Ala.	1,803	0.157	n.a.	n.a.	n.a.

Source: See appendix.
Note: n.a., not available.

had about 40 to 50 percent of local black households connected to public water and sewer lines. For a detailed explanation of how I "decluster" the original NMP estimates, see the appendix.

3.5 Conquering Waterborne Diseases and Improving Human Longevity

As table 3.4 shows, the total mortality rate in the United States fell by 39 percent between 1900 and 1940. The goal of this section is to estimate the proportion of this decline that can be attributed to the construction of public water and sewer systems, and the associated reductions in waterborne disease rates. The estimate is based on the assumption that waterborne diseases were eliminated solely through

Table 3.4
Reductions in Mortality: All Causes and Waterborne Diseases

Year	Deaths per 100,000 from		Percentage waterborne
	All causes	Waterborne diseases	
1880	1,509.1	146.4/186.7	0.096/0.124
1890	2,243.1	257.4	0.114
1900	1,755.0	169.1	0.096
1910	1,468.0	143.9	0.098
1920	1,472.1	57.5	0.039
1930	1,132.1	33.6	0.030
1940	1,076.4	13.3	0.012

Sources: U.S. Bureau of Census, *Census*, 1880, 1890, and 1900, various volumes and Linder and Grove, *Vital Statistics*, pp. 275–331.
Note: In 1880 typhoid was diagnosed with much less accuracy than in later years. The range in estimates reported for waterborne diseases reflects this. The lower-bound estimate ignores the tendency of doctors during this early period to conflate typhoid with malaria. The upper-bound estimate counts malaria as a waterborne disease. In chapter 7, I show that it is proper to treat malaria as a waterborne disease and that most deaths attributed to malaria in urban areas were probably typhoid.

improvements in public water and sewer systems. The analysis in chapter 2 suggests that this is a reasonable assumption.

There are two parts involved in estimating the benefits of eradicating waterborne diseases. The first part involves measuring the direct benefits of eradication and the second involves measuring the indirect benefits. To be precise, the phrase *direct benefits* refers to reductions in mortality resulting exclusively from reductions in waterborne diseases. The phrase *indirect benefits* refers to reductions in mortality resulting from reductions in diseases and health problems not specifically waterborne, but likely to be generated by exposure to typhoid. That is to say, estimating the indirect benefits involves measuring the frequency with which typhoid killed people slowly and indirectly, perhaps by inducing heart disease or pneumonia.

Estimating the direct benefits is straightforward. As table 3.4 shows, had you lived in 1890 or 1900, the odds that would you would have died from diarrhea or typhoid were very high; at the time, 1 out of every 10 Americans perished from these diseases. A half century later, the odds had much improved; by 1940, only about 1 out of every 100 Americans died from typhoid or diarrheal diseases. In short, between 1900 and 1940 the mortality rate from waterborne diseases fell by 92 percent, and deaths from waterborne diseases were largely eliminated.[17] Some simple math demonstrates that nearly one-quarter of the reduction in total mortality can be directly attributed to this dramatic reduction in waterborne disease rates. To see this, note that waterborne diseases represented about 10 percent of all deaths in 1900 and that the death rate from waterborne diseases fell by 92 percent. This implies that overall mortality fell by 9.2 percent as a direct result of the decline in waterborne diseases. Dividing 9.2 by the reduction in total mortality rates (39 percent) yields 24 percent.

Estimating the indirect benefits is more involved and much less precise. To get at the indirect benefits, it is first necessary to have some idea of incidence (i.e., the number of people falling ill from a specific disease in a specific population during a specific period). Incidence figures establish just how pervasive waterborne diseases were in turn-of-the-century American cities. In the case of diarrhea, a sample of records for nearly 35,000 Union Army soldiers suggests that around 1900, about one-third of all adult Americans suffered from chronic diarrhea. Complaints about diarrhea were so common and severe that doctors administering veterans' pension benefits developed a coding system to rank how disabling the ailment was.[18]

In the case of typhoid, incidence rates can be estimated. As stated earlier, typhoid fever itself killed only 5 to 10 percent of its victims; the remaining 90 to 95 percent survived the disease, at least in the short term. As shown in table 3.5, this implies incidence rates that are 10 to 20 times greater than reported mortality rates. For typhoid, it is also useful to calculate the probability that an individual would have contracted the disease at any point in his or her life. Assuming an average life expectancy, the final column in table 3.5 reports the upper- and lower-bound probability estimates of contracting typhoid once during a lifetime. These estimates suggest that around the turn of the twentieth century, about 1 out of every 3 Americans would have had typhoid at some point in his or her life.

Given these estimates, it seems reasonable to assume that about half of the American population would have been exposed to either a chronic diarrheal disease or typhoid at one point in their lives. Of these, most would have survived their bout with diarrhea or typhoid, but even if they survived the disease in the short term, the studies cited and discussed in chapter 2 suggest these survivors would have faced elevated risks of heart disease and respiratory problems in later life. Moreover, as explained earlier, complications from typhoid often in-

Table 3.5
Probability of Contracting Typhoid Once in a (Typical) Lifetime

Year	Death rate (d) per 100,000	Implied incidence rate (i) per 100,000: $i = d/(1 - 0.9)$	Probability of contracting typhoid in any given year (p): $p = i/100,000$	Probability of contracting typhoid sometime in one's life (P): $P = p \times (e^0)$
Assumes typhoid's case fatality rate was 10 percent				
1890	51.0	510	0.0051	$(0.0051) \times (42) = 0.214$
1900	35.9	359	0.0036	$(0.0036) \times (47) = 0.169$
1910	22.5	225	0.0023	$(0.0023) \times (50) = 0.113$
1920	7.6	76	0.0008	$(0.0008) \times (54) = 0.041$
1930	4.8	48	0.0005	$(0.0005) \times (60) = 0.029$
1940	1.1	11	0.0001	$(0.0001) \times (63) = 0.007$
Assumes typhoid's case fatality rate was 5 percent				
1890	51.0	1019	0.0102	$(0.0102) \times (42) = 0.428$
1900	35.9	718	0.0072	$(0.0072) \times (47) = 0.337$
1910	22.5	450	0.0045	$(0.0045) \times (50) = 0.225$
1920	7.6	152	0.0015	$(0.0015) \times (54) = 0.082$
1930	4.8	96	0.0010	$(0.0010) \times (60) = 0.057$
1940	1.1	22	0.0002	$(0.0002) \times (63) = 0.014$

Sources: See text for calculations and the following for data: U.S. Bureau of Census, *Census*, 1890, and 1900, various volumes and Linder and Grove, *Vital Statistics*, pp. 275–331.

cluded kidney and liver problems, pneumonia, and tuberculosis. It is perhaps no coincidence that the large reductions in waterborne disease rates that occurred between 1900 and 1940 were also associated with sharp reductions in tuberculosis death rates for both blacks and whites. Between 1900 and 1940, black tuberculosis rates fell by 71 percent and white rates by 79 percent.[19]

Given these observations, one would like to obtain a precise answer to the question of how much higher the death rates from pneumonia, tuberculosis, and heart disease would have been if the death rates from typhoid and diarrhea observed in 1900 had prevailed in 1940. Unfortunately, given the current state of knowledge, it is not possible answer this question with any precision. But one crude way to get an idea of the magnitude of the indirect benefits of eliminating waterborne diseases is by looking at the work of early-twentieth-century public health experts. Around 1900, experts like William T. Sedgwick of the Massachusetts Institute of Technology and Allen Hazen argued that purifying water supplies not only reduced deaths from waterborne diseases as narrowly defined, but also reduced deaths from diseases that did not immediately appear to have been waterborne (such as heart disease and tuberculosis). Sedgwick, Hazen, and others maintained that for every death from typhoid there were two to four additional deaths from such causes as pneumonia, tuberculosis, or heart disease. According to public health officials at the time, these additional deaths were ultimately caused by impure water, even though doctors had listed the cause of death as an illness that would not otherwise have been considered waterborne. This rule became known as the Hazen theorem or the Mills-Reincke phenomenon. As an illustration of the Hazen theorem, suppose that purifying the water supply of a particular city reduced the death from typhoid fever in that city from 100 to 10 deaths per 100,000 persons. Hazen's theorem implies that the death rate from all nontyphoid causes would have fallen by 180 (2 × 90) to 360 (4 × 90) deaths per 100,000 persons as a result of water purification.[20] As shown in table 3.6, Hazen's theorem suggests that about 20 percent of the decline in mortality observed between 1900 and 1940 can be attributed to construction of public water and sewer systems and the associated eradication of waterborne diseases.

Table 3.6
Hazen's Theorem and the Role of Pure Water in the Decline in American Mortality

	Rate	Hazen's multiplier			Total mortality rate
		2-1	3-1	4-1	
Calculations using typhoid fever rate					
1900	31.3	93.9	125.2	156.5	1,719.1
1940	1.1	3.3	4.4	5.5	1,076.4
Point reduction	30.2	90.6	120.8	151.0	642.7
(Change in typhoid rate)/(change in total mortality rate)	0.047	0.141	0.188	0.235	
Calculations using typhomalaria rate					
1900	37.8	113.4	151.2	189.0	1,719.1
1940	1.1	3.3	4.4	5.5	1,076.4
Point reduction	36.7	110.1	146.8	183.5	642.7
(Change in typhomalaria rate)/ (change in total mortality rate)	0.057	0.171	0.228	0.286	

Sources: See tables 3.4 and 3.5.
Note: Rate is deaths per 100,000 persons.

3.6   Implications for African-American Longevity

In the following sections of this chapter I provide some preliminary evidence to support my proposition that the construction of public water and sewer systems had especially large effects on the mortality rates of African Americans; further evidence is provided in subsequent chapters. For the time being, I focus on explaining why disadvantaged socioeconomic groups, such as African Americans and foreign-born whites, had the most to gain from improvements and expansions in public water and sewer systems. The discussion is built on the arguments of historians like Clayton R. Koppes and William P. Norris, who argue that disadvantaged groups had the most to gain from the purification of public water supplies because these groups "found it more difficult to undertake private measures to protect themselves from the risk of typhoid fever than did better-placed people."[21] Similar arguments have been developed by historical demographers. Specifically, in a well-known book and a series of articles, Samuel H. Preston and multiple coauthors have explored the sources of improvements in infant mortality during the late nineteenth and early twentieth centuries.[22] Their research suggests that household behavior played an increasingly important role in disease prevention over the course of this period.[23]

To understand why improvements in public water and sewer systems might have had differential effects across racial groups, it is first necessary to understand the sorts of things that families and individuals could do, in the absence of any actions by public officials, to prevent waterborne diseases. They could do four things to prevent typhoid. They could test their water for bacterial contamination; they could purchase bottled water; they could boil their (tap) water before using it; and they could install household filters on their taps. Several factors, however, limited the efficacy of such practices. First, it was costly for individual households to test their water for contamination. It required a scientist trained in bacteriology to identify intestinal bacteria in water.[24] Second, bottled water was much more expensive than tap water. In 1920, tap water from public systems sold at 0.015 to 0.025 cent a gallon, while bottled water sold for 8 to 10 cents per gallon, or in other words, three to seven hundred times the price of tap water.[25]

Third, typhoid bacteria are resilient. They can live in ice, frozen solid for several months. Though sunlight eventually kills them, they can withstand heat up to 160°F. Dried on inanimate objects—clothes, knives, forks, and so on—they can survive for several months. In dust, sand, and dirt, the bacilli live for several weeks. Even washing tainted glasses or silverware with alcohol does not always kill typhoid bacilli. Such resiliency imposed a heightened level of cleanliness and care on the part of water consumers before public filtration and chlorination were instituted. In 1910, the typical American household consumed 20–40 gallons of water a day.[26] Although only a fraction of this water was used for cooking and drinking, the resiliency of typhoid bacilli meant that families would have needed to boil all of their water, whatever its use, to have been completely safe from the disease. As noted earlier, for example, there were cases where individuals were infected after consuming fruits and vegetables washed with typhoid-contaminated water.[27]

Finally, while household filters were effective in removing large mineral deposits from water and in providing an element of water softening, they were not effective in eliminating bacteria from water and in some cases could actually cause bacteria to proliferate. Most household filters attached to kitchen faucets and contained a porous stone. When the homeowner turned on the faucet, water flowed through the pores of the stone. In theory, this process was supposed to filter out objectionable material, including bacteria. Unfortunately, the holes in even the most finely pored stones were many times larger than even the largest bacteria, and most bacteria went through the filter untouched. Furthermore, those bacteria that did not get through often lodged themselves on the interior walls of the stone, where they stayed on, untouched by any efforts to clean the stone with a brush. These tiny, interior pores were an ideal breeding ground for bacteria, and once inside, the bacteria proliferated. Consider the description of an experiment conducted by the Florida State Board of Health:

During the past two years a number of determinations, to ascertain the merits of the household filter, have been made. A popular type of filter was tested. Jacksonville tap water with an initial bacterial count of 35 per cubic centimeter was filtered through one of the porous stone filters; filtered water had a count of 950 in one instance and over a million in another.[28]

The ability to prevent typhoid and other waterborne diseases would have varied according to income and education. Blacks and other poor socioeconomic groups did not have the resources to purchase expensive bottled water or acquire information on appropriate sanitary practices, such as boiling potentially contaminated drinking water. Consequently, if they could not acquire tap water from the local supplier, they would have had few alternatives other than using their own dubious well water. Whites, who were relatively wealthy and better educated, were in a better position to buy bottled water and to obtain information on preventive practices.

Largely because black schools were systematically underfunded by local governments, in 1900 nearly half of all blacks over the age of fourteen were illiterate. The illiteracy rate was 44 percent, seven times the illiteracy rate for whites (6.2 percent).[29] To the extent that literacy determined a household's ability to acquire information about how to best prevent disease, black families would have been severely disadvantaged relative to white families.[30] In a similar argument regarding immigrant populations in Pittsburgh, Pennsylvania, Koppes and Norris write: "Home remedies required good general health knowledge, which probably was harder for immigrants to acquire, especially if they did not speak English."[31]

This line of thought predicts that blacks would have benefitted more than whites from improvements in local water systems. Consistent with this prediction, a recent study shows that New Deal spending on rural water and sewer systems in the American South significantly reduced black infant mortality rates, but had a relatively small effect on white rates.[32] Moreover, evidence presented in the next two sections and in chapter 6 indicates that the installation of water purification systems for public supplies had a much larger effect on black typhoid death rates than on rates for whites.

3.7   A Case Study of Water Filtration in Pittsburgh

Pittsburgh had a truly awful public water system for much of the nineteenth and early twentieth centuries. Before 1908, the city had the highest typhoid rate of any major American city, and during the early 1900s the typhoid rate in Pittsburgh was 3.5 times greater than the average rate in comparable American cities. Pittsburgh's typhoid problem stemmed from the fact that the city drew its water from rivers polluted by untreated sewage, and the city did not begin treating or filtering the water until 1908. Pittsburgh also lagged in its construction and installation of sewers. As of 1890, less than 20 percent of all homes in Pittsburgh were connected to the local sewer system, which is well below the connection rate in the mean American city (0.34).[33]

Pittsburgh's poor water and sewer system affected African Americans and the foreign-born disproportionately. As table 3.7 shows, before filtration, blacks and foreign-born whites were two times more likely to have died of typhoid than native-born whites. Some authors attribute such disparities in disease rates to a failure of public authorities to install water and sewer lines in neighborhoods with large numbers of African Americans and foreign-born whites. (See section 3.3 for data on water purification in major U.S. cities and the discussion on Chicago and Philadelphia in chapter 2.) In contrast, Koppes and Norris argue that while blacks and immigrants might have had relatively limited access to public water lines, the primary cause of excessive typhoid mortality among these groups was the failure of the city to adequately filter the water it drew from the Monongahela and Allegheny rivers. The city's failure to filter its water adversely affected blacks and immigrants much more than native-born whites because poor socioeconomic groups were disadvantaged in their ability to use the household precautions necessary to prevent typhoid.[34]

There is a simple way to test these competing explanations. If blacks and foreign-born whites had little or no access to public water supplies, when the city began filtering this supply in 1908, typhoid death rates for whites would have dropped while the rates for blacks and the foreign-born would have been unaffected. On the other hand, if blacks and immigrants were disadvantaged in terms of their ability to prevent typhoid privately, filtration would have benefitted them more than native-born whites. Figure 3.3 plots typhoid death rates for blacks, foreign-born whites, and native-born whites in Pittsburgh from 1890 through 1920. The patterns shown here contradict the idea that blacks and immigrants had little or no access to public water supplies, and confirm the hypothesis that poor socioeconomic groups benefitted disproportionately from filtration. Black and foreign-born typhoid death rates plummeted immediately following the installation of the filter in 1908, and racial disparities in these rates were largely eliminated after 1908.

Figure 3.4 plots the difference between typhoid death rates for blacks and native-born whites and foreign and native-born whites. This figure highlights how dramatically racial disparities in these rates fell in the years following the installation of the water filter. The difference in typhoid death rates for blacks and native-born whites fell from a peak of 140 to about 10 immediately after 1908, and exhibited a downward trend in the following years. The difference between foreign-born and

Table 3.7
Typhoid Rates in Pittsburgh

Group	Before filtration		After filtration		Observed change		Net-of-trend change	
	N	Typhoid rate	N	Typhoid rate	Point	Percentage	Point	Percentage
African American	8	109.1	5	14.8	94.3	0.864	164.0	0.917
Foreign-born white	8	97.1	5	20.5	76.6	0.789	131.9	0.865
Native-born white	8	47.9	5	7.7	40.2	0.839	60.3	0.887

Sources: City of Pittsburgh, *Annual Report of the Department of Public Health* (earlier titles include *Board of Health*) all available years, 1888–1920 and U.S. Bureau of Census, *Mortality Statistics*, all years, 1900–1920.

Note: Rate is deaths per 100,000 persons.

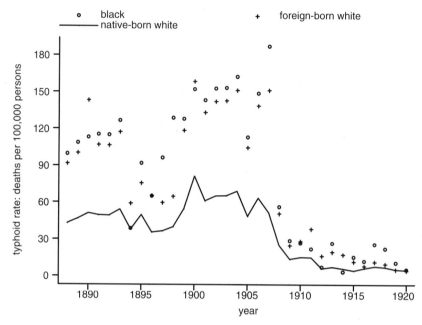

Figure 3.3
Race and typhoid death rates in Pittsburgh, 1890–1920. Typhoid rates are observed directly for native-born and foreign-born whites in 1890, 1894–1898, 1900, 1907, and 1911–1915. For blacks, typhoid rates are observed in 1890, 1894–1898, 1900, 1907, and 1911–1920. For other years, typhoid rates by race are inferred, using simple regression techniques, from data on overall typhoid rates. Sources: City of Pittsburgh, *Annual Report of the Department of Public Health* (earlier titles include *Board of Health*) all available years, 1888–1920; and U.S. Bureau of Census, *Mortality Statistics*, all years, 1900–1920.

native-born whites also fell sharply, although not as much as the difference in the rates for blacks and native-born whites.

Table 3.7 reports more precise calculations of the effects of filtration across racial groups. Black typhoid death rates fell by 86 percent after filtration, from an average of 109 deaths per 100,000 persons during the prefiltration period to 14.8 after filtration. For foreign-born whites they fell by 77 percent, from an average of 97 deaths per 100,000 persons to 20.5. Typhoid rates for native-born whites fell by 84 percent, from 48 deaths per 100,000 persons to 8. Although the percentage reductions that resulted from filtration are qualitatively similar across racial groups,[35] there are large differences in the point reductions across groups; black typhoid death rates fell by 94 points and those for foreign-born whites by 77 points, while white rates fell by only 40 points. These patterns are consistent with the idea that poor socio-

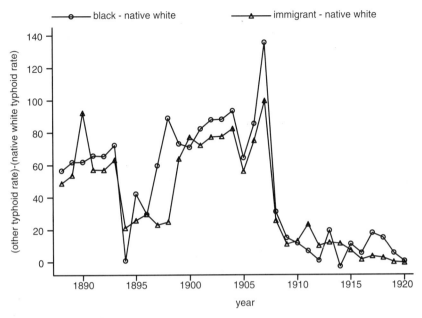

Figure 3.4
Racial disparities in typhoid and water filtration. Typhoid rates are observed directly for native-born and foreign-born whites in 1890, 1894–1898, 1900, 1907, and 1911–1915. For blacks, typhoid rates are observed in 1890, 1894–1898, 1900, 1907, and 1911–1920. For other years, typhoid rates by race are inferred, using simple regression techniques, from data on overall typhoid rates. Sources: City of Pittsburgh, *Annual Report of the Department of Public Health* (earlier titles include *Board of Health*) all available years, 1888–1920; and U.S. Bureau of Census, *Mortality Statistics*, all years, 1900–1920.

economic groups benefitted more than wealthier groups from the installation of water purification systems. Table 3.7 also reports the net-of-trend changes in typhoid death rates that resulted from water purification. In these calculations, prefiltration trends in typhoid death rates are used to predict what the rates would have been in the absence of filtration. Because these rates were trending upward before 1908, the net-of-trend changes are larger than the observed changes.

3.8   The Impact of Public Sewers on the Disadvantaged: Further Evidence

While we have discussed the role of income and education in determining the ability of persons in different socioeconomic strata to prevent disease at the household level, other factors may also have been operating that affected their health. It seems plausible that biological immunities to specific diseases also varied among ethnic groups. These differences could have arisen because of genetics or because of variation in the frequency (and type) of *in utero* insults in different populations. Simply put, in private efforts to battle typhoid, a given population could have been disadvantaged in its ability to alter its health-related behaviors, or persons in the population might have had immune systems that were compromised in some way. In this section I employ this broader notion of disadvantaged. I also offer statistical evidence that goes beyond the circumstantial evidence offered in section 3.7.

The data used here are the same as those used in chapter 2 to identify the effects that access to sewers had on infant deaths from diarrhea. Recall that these data come from a study of infant deaths in Baltimore, Maryland, where households were divided into cells according to their race, income class, and access to public sewers. With these data, the infant death rate from diarrhea is regressed against the infant death rate from nondiarrheal causes. These regressions are estimated separately for populations with and those without access to sewers. The infant death rate from nondiarrheal causes serves as a proxy for the "overall healthfulness" of the population. Those populations who were disadvantaged in some way (i.e., had low overall healthfulness) would have had high death rates from nondiarrheal causes. Those populations who were not disadvantaged would have had relatively low death rates from nondiarrheal causes.

Consider then the following regressions, run separately for cells with sewers and for cells without them:

Cells with sewers:

$$(\text{diarrhea rate}) = 0.012 + 0.106 \times (\text{nondiarrhea rate})$$
$$\quad\quad\quad\quad (3.00) \quad (1.01) \quad (t\text{-statistic})$$

$N = 24$, adj. $R^2 = 0.0006$ (Observations weighted by number of births in cell)

Cells without sewers:

$$(\text{diarrhea rate}) = 0.021 + 0.409 \times (\text{nondiarrhea rate})$$
$$\quad\quad\quad\quad (2.03) \quad (2.07) \quad (t\text{-statistic})$$

$N = 24$, adj. $R^2 = 0.1117$ (Observations weighted by number of births in cell)

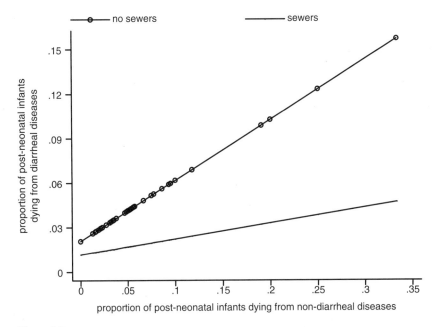

Figure 3.5
Overall healthfulness, diarrheal deaths, and access to public sewers. Circles indicate a
fitted relationship for cells (income and ethnic clusters) not connected to public sewers.
Straight lines indicate a fitted relationship for cells (income and ethnic clusters) connected
to public sewers. Source: See text.

These results indicate that among households with sewers, a variation in the death rate from nondiarrheal causes had little effect on the
diarrhea death rate. In contrast, among households without sewers, a
variation in the death rate from nondiarrheal causes had a much larger
effect—four times larger in fact—on the diarrhea death rate. The magnitude of the differential impact is illustrated graphically in figure 3.5.
Assuming that the death rate from nondiarrheal causes captures the
effects of the overall healthfulness of households, these results imply
that sewers gave homeowners room for health errors related to either
behavior or biology. Simply put, in households with public sewers,
people could forget to wash their hands or boil their water without
exposing their infant children to an increased risk of diarrheal disease.
Conversely, in the absence of sewers, health-related behavior and
natural immunities became much more important determinants of
infant health. Forget to wash your hands, boil your water inade-
quately, or have a compromised immune system, and the risk that

your infant child would die from diarrhea was increased fourfold over what households with sewers would have confronted.

3.9 Evidence from the Negro Mortality Project

The final source of evidence on the effects of public water and sewer systems on African-American health is the most direct. In particular, data from the Negro Mortality Project are used to identify the incidence of waterborne diseases among urban blacks and to identify how access to public water and sewer lines reduced these disease rates. The NMP data demonstrate that at the turn of the century, waterborne diseases were rampant among the African-American population and access to public water and sewer lines dramatically reduced the incidence of these diseases.

Table 3.8 shows the incidence of waterborne diseases among African-American populations surveyed by the NMP. As I explain in an appendix, these data are imprecise and based on the self-reporting of illnesses. With this caveat in mind, the table reveals three notable patterns. First, there is a high degree of intercity variation in incidence rates. In Washington and Birmingham, Alabama, 2–3 percent of the population reported having been sick from some type of a waterborne disease during the previous year, while in Sanford, Florida, more than a third of the population reported having had a waterborne illness. The following analysis demonstrates that this variation is driven largely by access to public water and sewer facilities. Second, the overall incidence of waterborne diseases appears to have been quite high. In the typical city, about 12 percent of the population reported having had a waterborne illness during the previous year. If the data are weighted by sample size, 8 percent of the sample reported having had a waterborne illness. Third, assuming a life expectancy of 30 years, this last statistic implies that the typical urban-dwelling black would have contracted a waterborne disease at least once in his or her lifetime. In terms of typhoid, the urban blacks surveyed by the NMP were three to five times more likely than whites to have been afflicted with the disease. The pervasiveness of waterborne diseases among African-American families at this time suggests that eliminating these diseases would have had a large effect on black longevity.

Figure 3.6 plots the incidence of waterborne disease in NMP neighborhoods[36] against the proportion of the population in those neighborhoods that had access to public water and sewer lines. This figure suggests a strong correlation between connections to public water and

Table 3.8
Incidence of Waterborne Disease among Households Surveyed by the NMP

	Proportion of population ill from			
	Diarrhea	Dysentery	Typhoid[a]	Total
Athens, Ga.	0.000	0.014	0.165	0.178
Atlanta, Ga.	0.002	0.002	0.059	0.062
Birmingham, Ala.	0.016	0.016	0.000	0.032
Cambridge, Mass.	0.008	0.000	0.025	0.033
Cartersville, Ga.	0.019	0.000	0.057	0.075
Chattanooga, Tenn.	0.000	0.000	0.034	0.034
Columbia, S.C.	0.000	0.000	0.222	0.222
Jackson, Tenn.	0.000	0.000	0.134	0.134
Jacksonville, Fla.	0.000	0.003	0.049	0.052
Louisville, Ky.	0.000	0.014	0.014	0.029
Macon, Ga.	0.000	0.011	0.167	0.178
Macon, Miss.	0.000	0.016	0.141	0.156
Nashville, Tenn.	0.006	0.001	0.061	0.067
Orangeburg, S.C.	0.000	0.000	0.110	0.110
Sanford, Fla.	0.000	0.000	0.371	0.371
Savannah, Ga.	0.000	0.000	0.142	0.142
Tuskegee, Ala.	0.000	0.000	0.067	0.067
Washington, D.C.	0.000	0.000	0.017	0.017
Average	0.004	0.004	0.106	0.115
Weighted average	0.003	0.002	0.076	0.080

Source: U.S. Department of Labor, "Condition of the Negro."
[a] Illnesses coded as malaria are counted as cases of typhoid. In chapter 7 I show that it is appropriate to treat cases of malaria as cases of typhoid because in nearly all cases illnesses diagnosed as malaria were in fact typhoid.

sewer lines and the incidence of waterborne disease. For neighborhoods where more than 30 percent of the population was connected, the incidence of waterborne disease never rose above 6 percent. In contrast, for neighborhoods where less than 30 percent of the population was connected, waterborne diseases were pervasive, and as many as 37 percent of all persons surveyed had been afflicted with a waterborne disease during the past year.

3.10 Summary

Three conclusions emerge from this discussion. First, cities were much less segregated in 1900 than they are today. Second, between 1900 and 1920, urban water and sewer systems were expanded with great

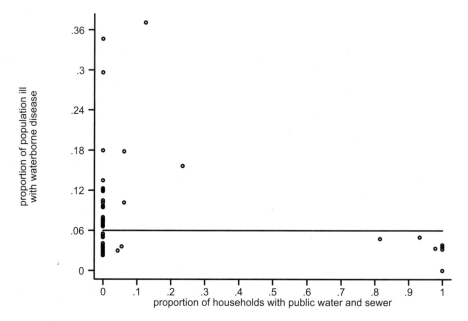

Figure 3.6
Access to public water and sewer lines and the incidence of waterborne disease in neighborhoods surveyed by the NMP. Source: U.S. Department of Labor, "Condition of the Negro."

speed, so that by 1915, half of all American cities estimated that they had connected more than 95 percent of their populations to public water supplies. While black neighborhoods appear to have received service with a lag, that lag was small—around 5 years—and might have had a legitimate policy rationale related to the fact that blacks tended to live in less densely populated areas. Furthermore, even before cities began rapidly expanding their water and sewer systems during the early 1900s, it was common for African-American families to have been connected to public water and sewer lines. For example, in Cambridge, Massachusetts, and Washington, D.C., about 90 percent of all African-American families were connected to public water and sewer lines. The third conclusion flows from the first two. Because water and sewer systems were built in an era of relatively low residential segregation, the networked structure of those systems made it difficult for local governments to build systems that did not adequately serve all populations, regardless of race.

Another issue addressed in this chapter is the role that the construction of water and sewer systems played in promoting human longevity. It is estimated that about 20 percent of the decline in human mortality observed between 1900 and 1940 can be attributed to the construction of public water and sewer systems, and the associated elimination of waterborne diseases. African-American households appear to have benefitted disproportionately from improvements in public water and sewer systems. Systematic evidence of disproportionate benefits is presented in chapter 6, but the case study of Pittsburgh presented above is, by itself, strongly suggestive. Why did blacks benefit disproportionately from improvements in public water and sewer systems? Because social obstacles hindered their ability to prevent waterborne diseases through private action. For example, discrimination in labor markets limited black economic progress and made it difficult for blacks to purchase purified and disease-free bottled water, which was much more expensive than tap water.

4

Typhoid Mary Meets Jim Crow: Stories from Memphis, Savannah, and Jacksonville

4.1 Introduction

This chapter describes the development of water and sewer systems in Memphis, Tennessee; Savannah, Georgia; and Jacksonville, Florida. Memphis, the site of the worst epidemic in American history, provides a natural setting in which to explore the role disease played in the construction of water and sewer systems. Savannah, like Memphis, experienced severe yellow fever epidemics, but unlike Memphis, did not respond to these epidemics in an equitable or aggressive manner in terms of extending its water and sewer systems. The chapter ends with an analysis of the rhetoric and ideology of Dr. C. E. Terry, the municipal health officer for Jacksonville, Florida. Terry's views on race and public health show how racial animus motivated white officials to extend water and sewer service to African-American neighborhoods.

4.2 Yellow Fever and the Miasmatic Theory of Disease

After the Civil War, the single most important event in nineteenth-century Memphis was the yellow fever epidemic that struck the city in 1878. Killing 1 out of every 8 Memphis residents, this was the worst epidemic (of any disease) ever to strike an American city.[1] As the epidemic raged during the summer, one-third of the black population and two-thirds of the white population fled the city. Of the blacks that remained in the city, 80 percent eventually contracted yellow fever; of these, 10 percent died. Of the whites that remained in the city, 98 percent eventually contracted yellow fever; of these, 70 percent died.[2] As its name implies, yellow fever adversely affects liver function (resulting in jaundice) and causes a high fever. Other symptoms include headache, restlessness, chills, and nausea. For those who survive, the disease reaches its peak 3 or 4 days after the onset of symptoms. For those who do not, the disease eventually causes kidney failure and internal hemorrhaging that manifests itself in blackened vomit and bleeding from the nose and mouth.[3]

To nineteenth-century observers, yellow fever was a mysterious disease. Unlike other major killers of the time, such as tuberculosis and typhoid, yellow fever killed more whites than blacks.[4] The disease would also lay dormant for years and then erupt suddenly, killing hundreds or thousands of people. In Memphis, for the half-century preceding 1878, in only 3 years (1855, 1867, and 1873) did anyone in the city die of yellow fever.[5] The disease's true transmission mechanism— the mosquito—was not discovered until the 1890s, and scientists did not reach a consensus on this issue until the early 1900s.[6]

By 1880, two schools of thought dominated the debate over the origins of yellow fever in particular and disease in general. Contagionists believed that yellow fever was spread by direct human contact. In many cities it was known as "stranger's disease," because it would appear suddenly and spontaneously, as though spread by some random stranger.[7] In contrast, anticontagionists believed that yellow fever originated in decaying matter and filth, and could be affected by climatological variables such as wind speed and direction, temperature, and rainfall.[8] According to anticontagionists, sewer gas was a poisonous agent that could, and often did, make people sick. Writing in 1879, a public health official in Georgia argued that "modern science has proven beyond refutation, that the germs of such diseases as yellow fever, typhus, and typhoid fever" were caused by the "putrefactive fermentations" of decaying human fecal matter.[9] During the early 1900s, some public health experts were still claiming that sewer gas killed thousands of people annually.[10] For the wealthy, the implications of anticontagionist interpretations of disease were no less frightening than contagionist interpretations. Disease-carrying poisons could develop amidst the squalor of poor neighborhoods, only to be spread to wealthy neighborhoods with the right gust of wind; in the case of yellow fever, it was even believed that poisons could be trapped inside the letters and luggage of infected persons and transferred to new places through such articles.[11]

To those who knew Memphis in 1878, such elastic interpretations of yellow fever must have made some sense. The city's climate—hot and wet—seemed conducive to the proliferation of miasmatic poisons; the disease appeared to arise spontaneously, as though spread by the wind or some new arrival to the city; and by most accounts Memphis was a filthy place. There were only a few miles of private sewers and most residents dumped their waste in privy vaults or in open ditches that flowed into nearby bayous. There was no system of stormwater drainage or public garbage disposal. Except for a small, poorly run private company, there was no public water supply; 72 percent of the city's 4,744 private wells used for drinking water were within 50 feet of privy vaults and were most likely contaminated by human waste. Hundreds of buildings in the city had standing water 2 to 18 inches deep in their basements or cellars; and the few city streets that were not dirt were made of rotting wood that emitted a foul smell. Even the city's own newspaper conceded that "all visitors" saw Memphis as "the filthiest and most deathly appearing town in the Union."[12]

Believing that all of this filth had something to do with yellow fever, officials in Memphis launched a massive campaign to cleanse the city of disease-causing fomites and poisons. In the midst of the epidemic, officials hired teams of blacks to empty all the privy vaults and disinfect them with carbolic acid. The wastes of yellow fever victims were then to be treated with acid and disposed of in impervious containers. The towels, blankets, sheets, curtains, furniture, and mattresses of yellow fever victims were washed with carbolic acid; when these items were too soiled to be cleaned, they were burned. Hundreds of houses so unsanitary that they were suspected of harboring poisons were burned. Mail entering and leaving the city was fumigated. Trains and boats entering and leaving the city were quarantined, as were their passengers. Refugee camps were set up outside the city and large fires were burned at night to disinfect the air.[13]

By the time the epidemic subsided in the winter of 1879, the city was bankrupt. After revoking the city's charter, the state also stripped Memphis of its name. The city was now referred to as "The Taxing District of Shelby County." On January 1, 1880, the population of the city formerly known as Memphis stood at 30,659, three-quarters of its population in 1870 (40,226). But taxes were raised and the cleaning continued.[14]

4.3   Building the Memphis Sewer System

The most significant and lasting manifestation of the effort to cleanse the city was the Memphis sewer system. To design and construct the new sewer system, city officials hired Colonel George E. Waring, a

flamboyant and self-promoting engineer. Officials chose Waring for
two reasons. First, he fervently believed that sewer gas and soil contaminated by human fecal matter were the repositories of poison and
disease. Most Memphis leaders shared this view. Second, Waring
advocated the construction of separate sewer systems; that is, separate
systems for sanitary disposal and stormwater drainage. The primary
appeal of the separate sewer system was its cost; it was cheap. Constructing a sanitary sewer system alone and using ditches and gutters
to drain off excess water saved thousands of dollars, a nontrivial consideration for a bankrupt city.[15]

The system Waring designed for Memphis was a model of economy.
The pipes were small; there were few manholes; and there was limited
capacity for dealing with overflows. To clean the sewers, gravity was
used to draw water from 112-gallon flush tanks through the sewer
mains. Because gravity was central to the operation and drainage of
the sewers, the following low-lying areas of Memphis were excluded
from the system: parts of South Memphis (the southernmost area of the
city); Chelsea (the northernmost area of the city); and land in the valley
on either side of the Bayou Gayoso. Sewering these areas would have
required the construction of a separate system of mains or the installation of pumps to flush the mains. Rejecting these options as too expensive, city officials decided that in areas that were not immediately
sewered, residents would be required to fill in their privy vaults and
install earth closets. An earth closet was an iron box buried beneath a
privy seat; the box had handles to ease removal and cleaning. In contrast to privy vaults, which were often little more than holes in the
ground, earth closets were watertight and did not allow their contents to pollute nearby soil or water sources. In theory, the contents
of earth closets were to be gathered by scavenger services that would
sell them to neighboring farms for fertilizer or dispose of them in the
Mississippi.[16]

Not all residents reacted positively to the economy of the Waring
sewer system. In a particularly revealing letter to the Memphis *Daily
Appeal*, a local doctor argued that the poor could not be trusted to clean
and empty their earth closets properly:

Nothing will be easier under such a lax system than for the poor people, both
white and black, to empty those vessels upon the surrounding surface. This
will be convenient and you will never detect them and if you could, what
would you do with them? Fine them? They have nothing to pay. Put the men
and women on a chain gang?[17]

The doctor predicted dire public health consequences: "The alleys, streets, and commons will give rise to fetid gases never known in the history of the city. And if filth is an important factor in the production of ... yellow fever, then look out for a stampede next summer."[18] To address this concern, the city set aside funds to pay for the regular cleaning and emptying of earth closets. All homeowners, however, whether they lived in areas to be sewered or not, bore the cost of cleaning and backfilling existing privy vaults.[19]

Despite objections, construction of the Waring sewer system began in January 1880. Teams of men worked throughout the city installing mains. In 1880 alone, 25 miles of mains were installed. By 1884, the system Waring had originally designed was complete and included roughly 40 miles of mains. Within a decade, the city had also built separate sewer systems in Chelsea and South Memphis. As anticipated, installing sewers in these areas was difficult and costly. The city engineer in charge of the Chelsea system described the installation of one large lateral main:

[The installation of the main] was through very treacherous ground, water being very near the surface. Through a large portion of the distance the trench had to be braced to prevent caving, and the sewer pipe had to be kept up with each day's work, so as to drain the ground for the next day, water in the wells on the adjacent property standing within ten feet of the surface.[20]

Problems like this meant that mains associated with the Chelsea system were laid at an average depth of 9.25 feet, while mains associated with the system installed by Waring were laid at an average depth of 7.25 feet. In 1890, mains in Chelsea (including labor and materials) cost 84 cents per foot, 35 percent more than mains in higher parts of the city.[21]

4.4   Who Got Sewers in Memphis?

To assess the degree to which the Memphis sewer system underserved African Americans, data from the Integrated Public Use Micro Data Series (IPUMS) are combined with a map of the Memphis sewer system as of 1884. Constructed by historians at the University of Minnesota, the IPUMS data are based on a random sample of all respondents to various U.S. censuses. Because the 1880 census recorded the address and race of respondents, it is possible to determine the race and location of 1 percent of all Memphis families as of 1880 in relation to the location of sewer mains. For the discussion that follows, an address is

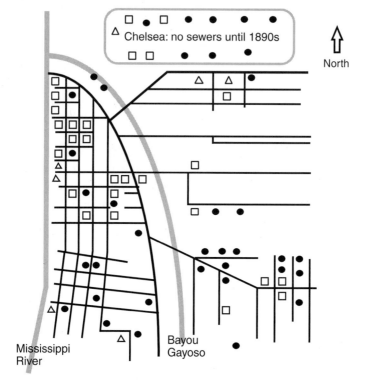

Figure 4.1
Memphis, Tennessee, sewer system in 1884. ▪ ▪ ▪, no sewerage until 1890s, including Chelsea and the area surrounding the Bayou Gayoso; □, white dwelling; ●, black dwelling; △, multirace dwelling. Scale: 1 inch equals approximately 2,000 feet. Sources: Tennessee State Board of Health, *First Report* (insert); Waring, *Sewerage*, pp. 114–23 (insert); and IPUMS, 1880 sample.

said to have had "access" to a sewer if it abutted a street or alley with a sewer line. While we cannot know for certain if abutting home-owners connected their dwellings to the sewer system, a city ordinance required all occupied houses along sewer lines to be properly con-nected to the line. Violators could incur a fine up to $50 (roughly $750 in 1991 dollars).[22]

The results are presented in figure 4.1. The map has been con-structed to maximize readability and is intended only to convey the broad contours of the sewer system and the location of different racial groups.[23] Thick black lines show the approximate location of sewer mains installed by the end of 1884. Shading indicates the two major areas in Memphis that went without sewers until the 1890s: Chelsea (the northernmost area on the map) and the land surrounding the Bayou Gayoso. The approximate locations of addresses occupied by blacks, whites, and multiple races as of 1880 are also shown. The racial patterns in residential location revealed here are consistent with previous historical studies. While patterns of segregation had already started to emerge in 1880, they were much less pronounced than a twentieth-century observer would expect; and to the extent there was segregation, blacks were concentrated on the periphery of the city and whites in the center of the city.

As the map illustrates, the sewer system reached the majority of population, whether black or white. Of the 78 addresses from the IPUMS sample, 78 percent had access to a sewer. Moreover, differences in rates of service across race were small and the majority of black-occupied addresses had access; 86 percent of white-occupied addresses had access to sewers and 72 percent of black-occupied addresses had access. If one excludes Chelsea residents from the IPUMS sample, 93 percent of all addresses, whether occupied by whites or blacks, had access. Indeed, almost the entire difference in access to service can be explained by the fact that blacks were more likely than whites to have lived in Chelsea; 20 percent of all black and mixed-race addresses were located in Chelsea; 14 percent of all white addresses were so located.

The failure to provide Chelsea, a majority-black neighborhood, immediate sewer service prompts the question of whether a similarly situated neighborhood that was mostly white have been treated the same way. The excuses offered by the city—the land was too low, the ground too wet—sound remarkably similar to the excuses white politicians offered when they refused to build, desegregate, and adequately fund black parks, schools, and public facilities. For the sake of argument, assume that the refusal to lay sewers in Chelsea was motivated purely by racial animus and that Memphis officials did not want to spend funds on a neighborhood that was primarily black. If white voters in Chelsea had any political power, this mode of discrimination would have imposed significant costs on local politicians. Based on the IPUMS sample, 46 percent of all Chelsea residents were white and were not disenfranchised by Jim Crow. This analysis suggests that discrimination in the provision of water and sewer systems was costly to white politicians and voters in a world with imperfect segregation because denying blacks service also required that whites be denied service.

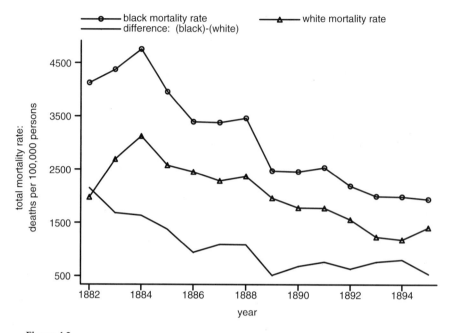

Figure 4.2
Total mortality rates in Memphis, 1882–1895. Source: U.S. Department of Labor, "Condition of the Negro," pp. 280–81.

Regardless of what motivated Memphis officials to delay bringing sewers to Chelsea, their construction benefitted both blacks and whites. Between 1884 and 1895, the total mortality rate (deaths from all causes per 100,000 persons) for both blacks and whites in Memphis fell by about 50 percent, and the difference between black and white death rates fell by about 70 percent (see figure 4.2). Looking exclusively at waterborne illnesses (cholera, diarrhea, and typhoid fever), the diseases most likely to have responded to the construction of sanitary sewers, the same conclusion emerges. Waterborne disease rates for both blacks and whites fell by about 70 percent between the early 1880s and the mid-1890s (see figure 4.3). These patterns contrast sharply with the way historians usually portray the distributive effects of the Memphis sewer system. Emphasizing the city's delay in bringing sewers to Chelsea, previous studies suggest that the primary beneficiaries of the sewers were middle and upper-class whites and that African Americans gained relatively little.[24]

By 1890, Memphis had one of the most developed sewer systems in the United States. According to the U.S. Census Bureau's *Social Statis-*

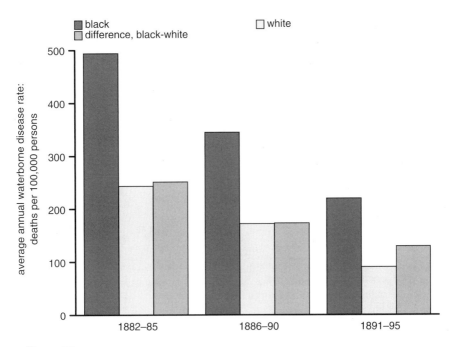

Figure 4.3
Mortality rates from waterborne diseases in Memphis, 1882–1895. Source: U.S. Department of Labor, "Condition of the Negro," pp. 280–81.

tics of Cities (1890), Memphis ranked among the top 10 or 15 percent of all U.S. cities in terms of the proportion of homes connected to the local sewer system, the top 20 percent in terms of miles of sewers per 10,000 persons, and the top 5 percent in terms of miles of sewers per 100 acres of land (see table 4.1).[25] Moreover, the data show that there were only small racial disparities in access to public sewer mains and that blacks benefitted as much, if not more, than whites in terms of disease reduction. What motivated Memphis officials to construct such a large and inclusive sewer system? Given the history described here, the answer seems obvious; it was fear of disease, particularly yellow fever. But like most obvious answers, this one requires qualification. Yellow fever alone cannot explain the intercity variation in the extensiveness of sewer systems. Other major southern cities, such as Baltimore, Maryland; Jacksonville; New Orleans, Louisana; and Savannah, also experienced yellow fever epidemics yet were very slow to develop and maintain adequate sewer systems.

Table 4.1
Sewer Systems in American Cities, 1890

	Proportion of all homes connected to sewers	Miles of sewer mains per 10,000 persons	Miles of sewers per 100 acres
Mean	0.340	6.77	0.580
Median	0.246	5.79	0.385
80th percentile	0.605	9.71	0.883
85th percentile	0.734	10.8	1.02
90th percentile	0.834	12.7	1.23
95th percentile	1.00	15.4	1.90
Memphis	0.812–0.882[a]	9.74	1.92
Savannah	0.499	3.70	0.426
Pittsburgh	0.179	3.65	0.501
No. of observations	126	207	207

Sources: Elliot, *Memphis Sewer System* and U.S. Bureau of Census, *Social Statistics of Cities*, 1890. Data prepared by Center for Population Economics, University of Chicago.
[a] Exact measures of the proportion of all homes connected to the Memphis sewer system as of 1890 are not available. The estimated range reported here has been constructed with data from Elliot, *Memphis Sewer System*.

4.5   A Counterexample: Savannah

Yellow fever epidemics struck Savannah in 1820, 1854, and 1876. Rivaling the Memphis epidemic of 1878, the 1876 epidemic killed as many as 1 out of every 13 Savannah residents who had not fled the city during the epidemic.[26] However, unlike Memphis, Savannah did not begin making major additions to its sewer system immediately; it waited 22 years. Savannah's slowness can be seen in table 4.1, which provides comparative measures of the development of the city's sewer system as of 1890. Although Savannah ranked above the mean American city in terms of proportion of homes connected to a sewer system, it ranked well below the mean in terms of miles of sewer mains per 10,000 persons and miles of sewer mains per 100 acres. Moreover, there is strong evidence that once Savannah authorities did respond to the threat of epidemic disease, they provided black neighborhoods with poorer service than white neighborhoods. In the discussion that follows, this can be seen directly by looking at maps of Savannah's water and sewer systems, and indirectly by analyzing how investments in water and sewer mains affected disease rates among blacks and whites. The following analysis indicates that segregated housing

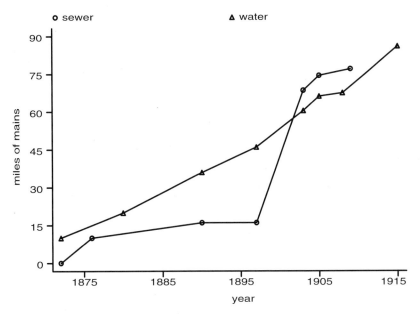

Figure 4.4
Miles of water and sewer mains in Savannah, 1872–1915. Sources: U.S. Bureau of Census, *Statistics of Cities*, 1905, p. 246 and *General Statistics of Cities*, 1909 and 1915, pp. 156–58; Baker, *Waterworks*, p. 356; Savannah, *Report of the Mayor*, pp. 320–56; U.S. Bureau of Census, *Social Statistics of Cities*, 1880, p. 173 and 1890. Data from U.S. census prepared by Center for Population Economics, University of Chicago.

patterns, which were more pronounced in Savannah than in Memphis, explain why Savannah authorities did not respond to yellow fever as vigorously or as equitably as those in Memphis.[27]

Figure 4.4 plots the development of the Savannah water and sewer systems from their inception in the mid-nineteenth century through 1915. Construction of the sewer system began in earnest in 1898, when the city installed over 30 miles of mains. The city had installed 69 miles of sewer mains by 1903 and 77 miles by 1909. Despite this growth, however, local authorities estimated that by 1909, only 62 percent of the city's population lived in homes connected to public sewers. In contrast to the sewer system, the Savannah water system grew steadily (see figure 4.4). By 1915, 86 miles of water mains had been installed and city authorities estimated that 95 percent of Savannah's population lived in homes connected to public water mains.

To assess the degree to which the Savannah sewer and water systems underserved African Americans, data from the public use samples are combined with maps of the systems that date from about 1900. The procedure here is identical to the procedure employed for Memphis, with one important exception. Because the IPUMS does not record the address of respondents from the 1900 census, the 1880 and 1920 samples (which do record addresses) are used to identify the racial makeup of specific addresses. A concern with this approach is that the location of black neighborhoods might have changed over time. To address this concern and to verify the location and racial makeup of specific Savannah neighborhoods, two historical sources are used to supplement the public use samples. The first source is the aforementioned Negro Mortality Project. The second complementary source is a historical survey of the city of Savannah conducted by the Federal Writers' Project during the 1930s, hereafter referred to as the FWP survey. The FWP survey focused exclusively on Savannah and resulted in a "historical walking tour" of the city. It enables one to locate, among other things, historically significant African-American churches, hospitals, neighborhoods, and schools.

Figure 4.5 shows the location of black and white households relative to sewer mains.[28] Sewer mains are identified with a bold line. Addresses occupied by at least one black are identified with a circle and addresses occupied solely by whites are identified with a square. Four predominately African-American areas that did not have access to sewers are highlighted and labeled 1–4. Both the NMP and FWP surveys indicate that the area labeled as 1 was known as Yamacraw, and describe it as an area with a predominantly African-American population. In the words of the FWP, "for the last century, this has been a Negro section of the city."[29] The NMP survey also suggests that the areas labeled 2, 3, and 4 correspond to predominantly African-American neighborhoods.[30]

Also, every African-American church, school, cemetery, and hospital that could be identified and located through the FWP survey is shown on the map. The Yamacraw neighborhood was home to the First Bryan Baptist Church. Founded by a slave who purchased his way out of bondage during the early 1800s, this structure remains a black church to this day. The first public school for blacks in Savannah was also located in Yamacraw. The church and school near neighborhood 4 were Saint Stephen's Episcopal Church and the Beach Institute. Founded in 1856, Saint Stephen's was the "oldest Episcopal Negro church" in Georgia. Founded in 1867 by the American Missionary Association and operated well into the twentieth century, the Beach Insti-

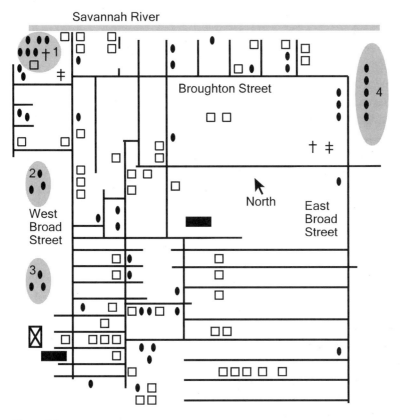

Figure 4.5
Location of black and white households relative to sewer mains in Savannah, 1900.
■ ■ ■, indicates predominantly black neighborhoods without sewerage circa 1900; □,
white dwelling; ●, black dwelling; other symbols: †, African-American churches; ‡,
schools; ⊠, cemetery; and ■■, hospitals. Scale: 1 inch equals approximately 1,500 feet.
Sources: U.S. Bureau of Census, *Social Statistics of Cities*, 1880; Savannah, *Report of the
Mayor*, pp. 360–72; FWP survey; NMP survey; and IPUMS, 1880 and 1920 samples.

tute was a private school for blacks and was located at the intersection
of Harris and Price streets. Located near the African-American neighborhood labeled as 3 were the Laurel Grove-South Cemetery and the
McKane hospital. Laurel Grove South was dedicated in 1852 and was a
black cemetery throughout the nineteenth century. The McKane hospital at 644 West 36th Street was founded in 1893 by a local doctor for
the care of black patients. Another black hospital, the Georgia Infirmary, was founded in 1832. But located at 1909 Lincoln Avenue (toward the center of the map), this infirmary was not in close proximity

to any of the black neighborhoods identified through the public use samples.[31]

Comparing the patterns of residential segregation observed in figures 4.1 and 4.5, it appears that segregation was more pronounced in Savannah than in Memphis. This finding is corroborated by standard indices of residential segregation: the dissimilarity index and the isolation index. These indices vary from 0 to 1, where 0 implies perfect integration and 1 implies perfect segregation. As of 1940, the first year that data are available for Savannah, the city's dissimilarity index equaled 0.710, which was 20 percent greater than Memphis's dissimilarity index (0.594). In the same year, Savannah's isolation index equaled 0.563, which was 30 percent greater than the isolation index for Memphis (0.432).[32]

Although the majority of black-occupied addresses in Savannah fronted streets with sewers, there is evidence that blacks were less likely than whites to have had access to the sewer system; 88 percent of white-occupied addresses fronted streets with sewer mains while only 59 percent of black-occupied addresses fronted such streets. Access to sewers was correlated with segregation; 81 percent (17 of 21) of black addresses that were without sewers were concentrated in the four neighborhoods identified as predominately black.

A map of Savannah's water system as of 1905 is presented in figure 4.6. A view of the water system 5 years after that of the sewer system, the map shows that water mains extended to nearly all inhabited portions of the city. Using the same coding procedure as earlier, by 1905 it is found that 100 percent of the households in the IPUMS sample, white and black, fronted streets with public water mains. Note, however, that the few inhabited portions of the city that were without water mains were located on Savannah's periphery and were most likely predominately black areas. This suggests that a handful of black-occupied addresses may not have fronted streets with water mains. In figure 4.6, the few inhabited areas without service are indicated by a light-gray shade.

Figure 4.7 plots the total mortality rate (measured as deaths per 100,000 persons from all causes) for blacks and whites in Savannah. Total mortality rates for both races rose between 1880 and 1900, dropped sharply after 1900, diverged (with white rates falling and black rates rising) after 1908, and started to reconverge after 1915. The sharp drop in black and white mortality immediately after 1900 coin-

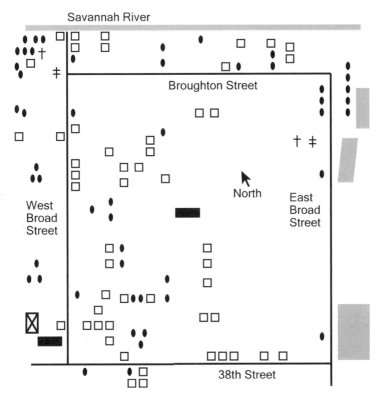

Figure 4.6
Map of Savannah's water system in 1905. ■ ■ ■, indicates areas without water service circa 1905; □, white dwelling; ●, black dwelling; other symbols: †, African-American churches; ‡, schools; ⊠, cemetery; and ▬, hospitals. Scale: 1 inch equals approximately 1,500 feet. Source: National Board of Fire Underwriters, *Savannah*; U.S. Bureau of Census, *Social Statistics of Cities*, 1880; Savannah, *Report of the Mayor*, pp. 360–72; FWP survey; NMP survey; and IPUMS, 1880 and 1920 samples.

cided with the rapid expansion of the sewer system, suggesting that sewers might have benefitted both races. However, whites appear to have benefitted more from such expansions since the difference between black and white mortality rose after 1905. It was only during the 1920s that this difference returned to the level observed 20 years earlier. As figure 4.8 shows, similar patterns emerge when one examines the behavior of waterborne disease rates over time. Again, the difference between black and white mortality showed no improvement until the 1920s, although black disease rates were falling over the entire period.

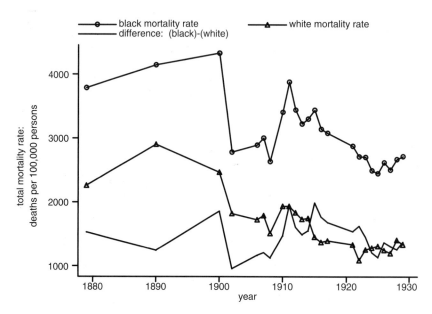

Figure 4.7
Total mortality rates in Savannah, 1879–1929. Sources: U.S. Bureau of Census, *Mortality Statistics*, various years; Savannah, *Report of the Mayor*, p. 20; U.S. Bureau of Census, *Census and Mortality Statistics*, 1890.

4.6   Jacksonville: Flies, Black Privies, and White Kitchens

During the early twentieth century, the municipal health officer for Jacksonville was Dr. C. E. Terry. In a series of papers delivered before the American Public Health Association, Terry developed the argument that poor hygiene and disease among African-American households undermined economic progress, and more important in the doctor's view, white health and longevity. Terry wrote:

The increase in the total death rate of our cities, through the excessive negro (sic) mortality, exerts a definite, harmful influence upon our growth and leads those, unacquainted with the facts, to erroneous impressions as to our sanitary standing. However rapid as has been the growth of many of our Southern cities during the past decade, through immigration from the North and West, I am convinced that, but for this deterring fact, it would have been still more rapid. This alone, however, is not worthy of passing consideration, in that it affects but the financial aspect of the subject. Of far greater import is, I believe, the direct influence of the negro race as a menace to our own—a source and disseminator of infection.[33]

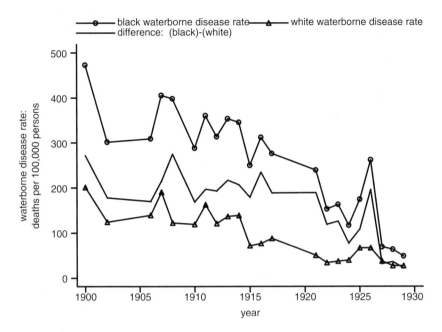

Figure 4.8
Waterborne disease rates in Savannah, 1879–1929. Sources: U.S. Bureau of Census, *Mortality Statistics*, various years, *Census and Mortality Statistics*, 1900.

According to Terry, the transmission vectors that connected black disease to whites were manifold, stemming from the fact that African Americans often worked as domestics and food handlers, cared for young white children, and worked side-by-side with whites in factories:

These negro citizens, amongst whom we find such an undue prevalence of diarrhoeal diseases, tuberculosis and venereal infections, who live under the worst of sanitary conditions, through circumstances of racial inferiority and our neglect, mingle with us in a hundred intimate ways, in our stores and factories, our kitchens and nurseries. They knead our bread and rock our babies to sleep in their arms, dress them, fondle them and kiss them; can anyone doubt that we may not escape this close exposure?[34]

Typhoid and related diseases represented yet another mode of disease transmission: "The missed and carrier cases of typhoid and other intestinal diseases that wait upon our tables must exact their toll nor is this lessened by any habits of personal cleanliness."[35]

However, for Terry, the transmission mechanism that posed the greatest threat to white health was the fly, which carried diseases from the open privies and unkempt homes of African Americans to the sewered and clean homes of whites. As Terry elaborated:

It must be remembered that for generations we have left this race to their own devices in their homes. They live for the most part in ill-ventilated shacks, without provision for sewerage or proper water supply. The privy, the surface well, the rain barrel and filthy stable are evidence of our own shortsightedness, and their needs.[36]

According to Terry, these conditions not only left blacks vulnerable to intestinal diseases such as typhoid and dysentery, they also left whites vulnerable, because in a world without sewers, flies interacted with the germs and wastes that African-American households deposited in open privies, and brought them to white homes: "Where, then, excretions from individual suffering from any of these maladies may lie exposed to the free access of flies it would seem that definite measures were necessary to prevent this exposure."[37]

To some extent, Terry spoke from experience. As the chief health officer of Jacksonville, he had observed firsthand conditions ideally suited for the spread of typhoid and dysentery by flies. Florida's climate encouraged the proliferation of flies, while Jacksonville's incomplete sewer system gave homeowners few options other than to dispose of human wastes in open surface privies. Moreover, it was not as though surface privies were concentrated in only one section of town; on the contrary, they were everywhere and homeowners with sewers were only a few hundred yards away from homeowners without them:

This surface-privy district is not confined to any one portion of the city but is distributed about evenly throughout every suburb and even in the older sections [of town]. In fact there is no point within the city limits of Jacksonville further than nine blocks from one or the other surface-privy district.... 75 percent of the population live within three or four blocks of surface privies, notwithstanding the fact that their own premises may have sewer connections.[38]

Terry's experiences in Jacksonville compelled him to rebuke colleagues who did not share his convictions about flies as a source of disease transmission:

In spite of the statement of Dr. Chapin that, "There is no evidence ... that the house fly is a factor of great moment in the dissemination of disease," I believe that, throughout the South at least, this insect plays an important role in such dissemination. In making this statement Dr. Chapin probably has in mind the well-sewered cities of the North. Jacksonville, like many other Southern cities, is not a well-sewered city.[39]

Conditions in Jacksonville were so foul that Terry drew the following unfavorable comparison between the city and an army camp:

Not only do the conditions of an army camp prevail in nearly every district [of the city], but I am inclined to believe that ... our conditions are worse than those of the average army camp where, at least, latrines are segregated to a certain section more or less remote from tents.[40]

And Terry went on to explain in graphic terms that were probably not unwarranted:

With us there are 8,500 privies impartially distributed throughout the city, each an open, reeking mass of excrement; each within twenty-five or thirty feet of an unscreened kitchen or dining room, and this in a climate where fly-breeding progresses unchecked by temperature for at least nine months in the year. Could any conditions be found more ideally adapted to fly carriage of infection?[41]

Coming from a man prone to hyperbole and incapable of transcending the bigotry of his time and place, Terry's arguments and factual claims deserve scrutiny. For example, Terry stated that the sewerage system did not cover "more than two-thirds of [Jacksonville's] population at most."[42] Yet the *General Statistics of Cities* reports that 75 percent of Jacksonville's population was connected to public sewers by 1909, 3 years before Terry delivered his paper. With 75 percent of its households connected to the public sewer system, Jacksonville was slightly below the median city in the North, and slightly above the median city in the South in terms of sewer connections. (For more data on access to sewers across cities, see table 3.1.)

At one point Terry strongly implies, although he does not expressly state, that nearly all African-American households in Jacksonville were without access to sewers.[43] This is incorrect. Survey data from the Negro Mortality Project suggest that as early as 1897, 35 percent of black households in Jacksonville were connected to public water and sewer lines.[44] It is also possible to construct a lower-bound estimate of access to sewers using data from the 1909 *General Statistics of Cities*. More than 50 percent of Jacksonville's residents were black, and 75 percent of all city residents were connected to public sewers (according to the *General Statistics*).[45] If we make the extreme assumption that 100 percent of all white households in Jacksonville were connected, this implies that no less than half of all African-American households were without sewers. And if the experiences of Baltimore, Maryland; Gary, Indiana; Savannah; and Memphis are any guide, this dramatically overstates the degree to which African-American households were underprovided relative to white households. (See chapter 3 for data on Baltimore and Gary.) Finally, Terry claimed that sewers in southern cities were much less extensive than those in northern cities. This too is incorrect. As shown in chapter 3, the North and South did not differ all that much in terms of the extensiveness of their sewer systems.

Nonetheless, Terry's broader argument that the failure to provide adequate public water and sewer services to black neighborhoods adversely affected white health had some foundation in fact, particularly his fear that flies contributed to disease rates in the city. During the early twentieth century, typhoid death rates in Jacksonville were among the highest in the nation. For example, between 1906 and 1910, the average American city had a typhoid death rate of 26.8 deaths per 100,000 persons; in Jacksonville over the same period, these rates averaged 155 per 100,000 persons, nearly six times the national average.[46] Jacksonville's problem with typhoid did not stem from impure water; the city drew its water from deep underground wells that were largely free from bacterial pollution. Instead, as explained earlier, the typhoid problem was the result of not having 100 percent of the city connected to public sewers. The quarter of the city's population that did not have sewers used surface privies to dispose of fecal matter. These privies attracted flies that crawled over the waste. When the waste was contaminated with typhoid (or any other diarrheal disease), the flies transmitted the disease to neighboring homes.

4.7   Exterminating Flies and Eliminating Typhoid

Partly in response to Terry's urging, Jacksonville authorities began taking steps to address the city's typhoid problem and to improve access to public sewers. In the short run, the most important of these steps was the passage of a public health ordinance in August 1910. This ordinance required that all unsewered households install flyproof screens on their privies. The ordinance also stated that anyone sick with typhoid had to be confined to a "sick room" in his or her home and that screens and flypaper must be used to prevent flies from carrying typhoid out of the room. In cases of financial hardship, the city agreed to furnish flypaper, netting, and screens free of charge. Terry claims that both provisions of the ordinance were vigorously enforced:

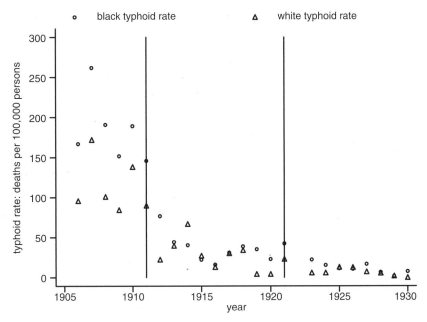

Figure 4.9
Black and white typhoid death rates in Jacksonville, 1906–1930. Vertical lines indicate the
implementation of the antityphoid ordinance in 1911 and the chlorination of the city's
water supply in 1921. Black typhoid rates include deaths from malaria. See chapter 7 for
an explanation of why malaria is included in black typhoid deaths. Sources: Florida State
Board of Health, *Thirty-Second Report*, 1922; U.S. Bureau of Census, *Mortality Statistics*,
various years; and Terry, "The Negro."

The enforcement of this ordinance was begun energetically, and by the first of
April [1911], between 80 and 90 percent of all privies had been reconstructed
according to its requirements. [By November 1911] probably 95 percent of
these [were] in good working order.[47]

As for the effective fly-quarantine of typhoid patients themselves,
Terry explained, "an inspector [is supposed to visit] each case every
other day from the time of its reporting until convalescence is
established."[48]

It appears that Terry's claims about "energetic enforcement" were
accurate. Figure 4.9 plots black and white typhoid death rates in Jacksonville from 1906 to 1930. The reduction after 1910 was dramatic, for
both blacks and whites. Between 1906 and 1910, black typhoid death
rates averaged 192 and white rates averaged 118 deaths per 100,000
persons; between 1910 and 1920, black rates averaged 43 and those for

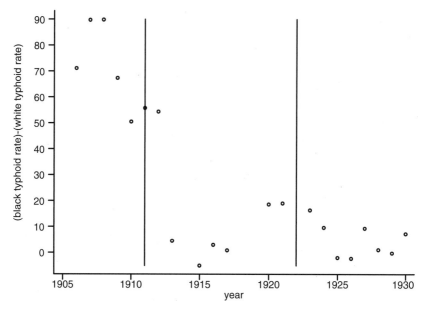

Figure 4.10
The difference between black and white typhoid rates in Jacksonville. Vertical lines indicate the implementation of the antityphoid ordinance in 1911 and the chlorination of the
city's water supply in 1921. Black typhoid rates include deaths from malaria. See chapter
7 for an explanation of why malaria is included in black typhoid deaths. Sources: Florida
State Board of Health, *Thirty-Second Report*, 1922; U.S. Bureau of Census, *Mortality Statistics*, various years; and Terry, "The Negro."

whites 33 deaths per 100,000 persons, a reduction of 78 and 72 percent,
respectively. There is mixed evidence that blacks benefitted disproportionately from this ordinance. Figure 4.10 shows that the difference between black and white typhoid rates fell from about 50 in 1910 to 4 in
1913, a reduction of 92 percent. However, figure 4.11, which plots the
ratio of black to white typhoid rates, suggests that blacks and whites
benefitted equally from the ordinance, with rates for both races falling
by about the same amount in percentage terms. Beyond this, it is notable that chlorination of Jacksonville's water supply, which began in
1922, had a much smaller effect on typhoid rates, in absolute terms,
than the antityphoid ordinance.

At least in the short run, Jacksonville's ordinance requiring that all
privies be made flyproof probably made more sense than immediately
laying sewer mains throughout the city. Even in cities that installed
sewers so that all households had access, there was often reluctance on

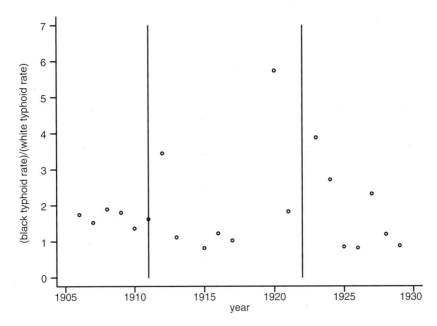

Figure 4.11
Ratio of black and white typhoid rates in Jacksonville. Vertical lines indicate the implementation of the antityphoid ordinance in 1911 and the chlorination of the city's water supply in 1921. Black typhoid rates include deaths from malaria. See chapter 7 for an explanation of why malaria is included in black typhoid deaths. Sources: Florida State Board of Health, *Thirty-Second Report*, 1922; U.S. Bureau of Census, *Mortality Statistics*, various years; and Terry, "The Negro."

the part of some households to connect to the lines. Around 1910, connecting to a sewer main could sometimes cost as much as $100. Rather than spending that much to connect to a sewer line, homeowners and landlords sometimes preferred to spend their money in other ways, in all likelihood to the great annoyance of their neighbors. Summarizing the evidence for Pittsburgh, for example, Joel Tarr writes:

While the Board of Health tried to mandate household connections to the sewers, both homeowners and landlords ... resisted, and retained their old privy vaults and cesspools. Even working-class homeowners often avoided connections with the sewer system because of costs, preferring to invest in other forms of home improvements.[49]

Because the cost of screening a privy was probably much lower than the cost of connecting to sewer lines, homeowners would have been much more likely to have undertaken the former approach.

4.8   Why Bigots Wanted Sewers for Everybody

It is important to be clear about what motivated Dr. Terry when he advocated extending water and sewer services to African-American neighborhoods. First, what did not motivate him was a genuine sense of equality and justice. His argument for installing water and sewer mains in African-American neighborhoods was not built on the idea that the races were equal or that as members of a common humanity they deserved the same level of service in this area of public health. Still, if Terry had based his arguments on such ideas, they probably would have had much less influence than they ultimately did. Terry was motivated by a mixture of naked self-interest—he did not want to be offended by the sight and smell of black privies, or risk diseases spreading from black privies to white households through flies or any other transmission mechanism—and a twisted sense of *noblesse oblige*—he wanted to help the members of an inferior race transcend their biological and cultural foibles by bettering the environment in which they lived. In Terry's own words:

Here, certainly, it would seem, is a field for new endeavor in modern sanitation. Aside from humanitarianism, we are confronted with the problem of self-protection, but as in all matters concerning public health, protection of others is a concomitant of self-protection. We may see a double result of labor expended.[50]

Whatever Terry's motivations, they were predicated on the view that blacks were incapable of helping themselves, and that only through the help of whites could they better themselves. Consider, for example, how Terry explained the inability of most African-Americans to get appropriate medical care:

We meet, here, one of the many contradictions in the mental equipment of the negro (sic). An alarmist by nature, where trifles are concerned, yet, in the presence of a truly grave condition, even with death at hand, his natural optimism prevents all foresight of a possible fatal termination.[51]

Only if whites intervened, according to Terry, could blacks come to appreciate the significance of proper health-related behaviors.

When Terry's arguments for improved sanitation are placed in the context of his racist ideology, it becomes clear that he advocated bringing water and sewers to black neighborhoods and households, not despite the race of the people who lived there, but because of it. More precisely, blacks needed public water and sewer facilities, not because they were the same as whites, but because they were inferior to them. In Terry's world view, a white man could be trusted with a privy; a black man could not. At one point Terry described "the most ignorant type of negroes" as "too lazy to support themselves in any manner," and "too ignorant" to fill out forms provided by government agencies or to abide by proper sanitary practices. Elsewhere Terry argued that "racial weakness will account for a percentage of the negro death rate above our own."[52] In the context of the fly-ridden South, how could a man like Terry trust a black man to put a screen on his privy and keep it there? The public health ordinance of 1910 was an adequate stopgap measure, but clearly, in the long run more drastic steps needed to be taken, such as the installation of public sewers.

Nor were Terry's views unique. Dr. William F. Brunner, the health officer for Savannah, developed a more extensive version of Terry's arguments in a paper he too presented before the American Public Health Association. According to Brunner, Terry understated his case. Like many other Progressive Era reformers, Brunner linked disease and poor health to moral decay, and so in his eyes, if left to their own devices, blacks would have not only transmitted diseases, they also would have promoted moral degradation:

The negro is with you all the time. He is what you will make him, and it is up to the white people to prevent him from becoming a criminal and to guard him against tuberculosis, syphilis, etc. If he is tainted with disease, you will suffer; if he develops criminal tendencies you will be affected.[53]

In short, "there is a contamination of the white race by the negro race and this contamination is both physical and moral."[54] How Brunner linked disease and moral decline can be seen in his analysis of tuberculosis and crowded housing conditions in Savannah:

The congestion of residences and of people in them is the one reason why, last year, 34 white people died of tuberculosis, and 124 negroes succumbed to that disease; and, for the same reason, 3 negro children die when 1 white child dies; and there are other diseases, causing a high death rate which are a result of this disregard of the laws of sanitation. The moral side figures here also. Would you expect an improved morality when families of male and female children grow up in direct contact which necessarily follows when the family is restricted to one room? Would you expect normal health conditions? It is time for the dominant white race to look this and kindred problems squarely in the face, and legislate for the betterment of these people.[55]

It is no accident that Brunner began his essay with a lengthy racist exposition about black history and how it purportedly demonstrated the inferiority of the race. Before exploring the significance of this passage, it is useful to document just how far it went. Brunner claimed that it was "certain" that blacks had helped build "Egyptian civilization," but only as "bearers of stone" and "carriers of water." It was also "certain" that once the building was completed, "the negro went back to the jungle and reverted to type." He went on to claim that after emancipation in the United States, "women and children began to raise the crops of rice, corn and potatoes, while the lords and masters worked a little and spent the rest of the time in hunting and fishing." Similarly, in describing settlement patterns among blacks in the postbellum South, Brunner wrote: "he was doing just what the dog does when he turns around several times before lying down."[56] Of course, none of this had anything at all to do with the topic at hand: African-American mortality in southern cities. But it did serve an important rhetorical end. Lest someone accuse Brunner of insufficient racial animus for advocating the extension of sanitary services to black neighborhoods, it served to tell the members of the audience: "Listen to me. I am one of you. I do not advocate these things because blacks are our equals; I advocate these things because they are our inferiors."

For Brunner, as for Terry, bringing blacks water and sewer was not inconsistent with racist ideologies of the day; on the contrary, it was the natural extension of such ideologies. Left to their own devices, blacks were incapable of surviving in a civilized way, and more important, their failings as a people would eventually, in Brunner's words, "contaminate" the white race, "physically and morally." So important was the influence of whites on blacks that Brunner even had a formula for the optimal number of blacks in any particular city:

He [the black man] is trying hard to become a good citizen and becomes a valuable asset provided that he is numerically not more than two-fifths of the community in which he lives. If he exceeds that percentage, his progress is retarded and, in a community where he greatly outnumbers the white population, he goes ahead not at all and furnishes a low morality and a high mortality. The cities of Wilmington, N.C., Charleston, S.C., Savannah, Ga., and Jacksonville, Fla., have an excess of negroes over whites and, therefore, each one of these cities is on a sanitary parity with the other.[57]

There is a clear parallel here between Brunner's idea that blacks could thrive only if they were surrounded by an adequate number of whites, and those of other nineteenth-century racists who justified various imperialistic enterprises through appeals to the "white man's burden." With such a paternalistic world view, Brunner could not help but advocate bringing improved sanitation such as water mains and sewers to black neighborhoods. It was like a religious conviction; blacks in urban America needed water and sewer lines as badly as blacks in Africa needed Christianity. Without the aid of whites, blacks would find neither salvation nor good health.

4.9 Conclusions

The experiences of Memphis and Savannah suggest three provisional hypotheses. First, there was intercity variation in the extent to which African-American neighborhoods received sewage and water services. Some cities, like Memphis, installed extensive and equitable systems that appear to have benefitted both whites and blacks; other cities, like Savannah, installed systems that benefitted whites but not blacks. Second, the experience of Memphis suggests that at least in extreme cases, fear of epidemic disease played a role in motivating cities to install relatively equitable sewer and water systems. Third, the experience of Savannah suggests that residential segregation facilitated efforts to underprovide African Americans with sewer and water services. In this way, the timing of the construction of water and sewer systems was critical. Because most cities and towns installed their water and sewer systems before 1920, during an era of relatively low residential segregation, it was difficult to construct systems that underserved African Americans without also underserving whites.

One caveat to the hypotheses just offered is that generalizing from the experiences of just two cities is difficult. For example, in terms of the overall access that African Americans had to sewer and water systems, it is not clear whether Savannah or Memphis had the more representative experience. A related objection is that the qualitative nature of the case studies makes it difficult to measure the relative and absolute importance of segregation and (fear of) epidemic disease in shaping the installation of sewer and water systems. Subsequent chapters, particularly chapters 6, 7, and 8, address these concerns.

The experience of Jacksonville highlights two important points. First, fly-related transmissions of typhoid could be significant in environments conducive to the proliferation of insects and in environments where sewer systems were incomplete. In the case of Jacksonville, it appears that fly-related transmissions of typhoid were effectively eliminated by an ordinance requiring households to screen their privies. This obviously was a much cheaper way of dealing with typhoid than installing sewer lines, although in the long run it probably would have been much less effective than installing sewers. Second, in contrast to other types of publicly provided goods, racism did not undermine the case for bringing black households water and sewer service. As Terry's words show, water and sewer lines for black households were imperative in a world where diseases were easily spread, and in a world where racist public officials like Terry believed that blacks were inherently lazy and careless.

5   The Exception That Proves the Rule: Shaw, Mississippi

5.1   The Case of *Hawkins v. Shaw*

More than thirty years ago, a group of African Americans living in Shaw, Mississippi, sued the town for violating their rights to equal protection guaranteed under the Fourteenth Amendment. According to the plaintiffs, the town of Shaw had discriminated against black neighborhoods when it provided public services, including sanitary sewers and water. As evidence of discrimination, the plaintiffs pointed to the following undisputed facts:

• Ninety-seven percent of all homes without access to sanitary sewers were occupied by blacks. While 99 percent of white homes had sanitary sewers, only 80 percent of black-occupied homes had sewers.
• Most white homes were served by 4- to 6-inch water mains, while most black homes were served by 1.25- to 2-inch water mains. Consequently, water pressure was much lower in black neighborhoods than in white neighborhoods.

Ruling against the city, a federal appeals court found that "no compelling state interests" could have "possibly justified" such patterns, and concluded that "a violation of equal protection had occurred."[1]

    Civil rights activists and legal observers hailed *Shaw* as a watershed decision. Writing in the *Harvard Civil Rights-Civil Liberties Law Review*, one commentator hoped that "by providing the first precedent for invalidating varying patterns of municipal services," *Shaw* would become "the progenitor of cases attacking the unequal provision of municipal services."[2] Another commentator characterized the decision as "revolutionary" and "brilliant," and predicted that *Shaw* would become as significant as *Brown v. Board of Education*.[3] And on its face, *Shaw* certainly appears to have been a case that was pregnant with implications for public policy; surely predictions that *Shaw* would rival *Brown* in terms of its historical and legal significance were not unfounded at the time. Moreover, the decision itself appears to have improved things in Shaw. Shortly after a federal court handed down the decision in 1971, city officials devised a plan to equalize access to public services in the town, and public services were expanded. Today, there are some new street lights, most streets have been paved, and new curbing has been installed. The open ditches that served as storm drains have disappeared, and new water and sanitary sewer mains have been installed so that today 97.5 percent of the town's homes have access to the sewer system, and 100 percent of homes have access to the public water system.[4]

Yet, when one goes beyond the confines of the town of Shaw, the broader significance of the case is much less clear. Despite predictions to the contrary, *Shaw* did not spawn a wave of similar lawsuits, at least with regard to access to public water and sewer lines. As explained later, since 1960 there have been only a handful of cases where cities were sued because they failed to provide African-American neighborhoods adequate water and sewer systems. Nor is there any evidence to suggest that *Shaw* had a significant impact on African-American access to public services in municipalities other than Shaw. After the decision was handed down, there was no nationwide integration of public water and sewer systems, as was the case with schools following *Brown*. And as for *Shaw* being the next *Brown*, evidence presented later shows that while subsequent legal decisions have cited *Brown* more than 9,000 times, *Shaw* has been cited fewer than 250 times. Although this is still a substantial number of citations, the decisions that cite *Shaw* typically have little to do with discrimination in the provision of municipal services and more to do with the evidentiary standard for discrimination articulated by the courts in *Shaw*, a standard that has since been overturned by the U.S. Supreme Court (see section 5.2).

This chapter explores the significance of *Shaw* by placing the decision in a broader historical and legal context. In doing this, it develops three arguments. The first is that the town of Shaw was a very unusual place and that it is not surprising that such a place would generate a legal ruling with little relevance for more typical American cities and towns. Shaw, for example, did not begin building a sewer system until 1963, even though it was located in a region subject to frequent flooding. The second argument builds on the following assumption: If African Americans were denied access to public water and sewer lines in the same way that they were denied access to public schools, the amount of litigation regarding access to public water and sewer facilities would be qualitatively similar to the amount of litigation on access to public education. The third argument uses comparisons of Shaw and the handful of other municipalities that have been found guilty of discriminating in the provision of these services.

5.2   Putting Shaw in Context

A History of Shaw

Located 20 miles east of the Mississippi River and 160 miles southwest of Memphis, Tennessee, Shaw is situated on the Mississippi Delta in Bolivar County, Mississippi. Like other towns on the Mississippi Delta, Shaw is flat, hot, wet, and subject to frequent flooding. From June through September the average daytime temperature exceeds 90°F. Average annual rainfall exceeds 50 inches. In addition, two bayous run through the town, which lies only 130 feet above sea level. Historically, the heat, flooding, and ever-present drainage problems in the delta encouraged the proliferation of disease-carrying mosquitoes. Consequently, malaria and yellow fever plagued the region throughout the nineteenth and early twentieth centuries. During the 1870s, yellow fever epidemics killed thousands. In 1900, malaria was the region's third leading cause of death. Only when public health authorities in the South began to install drainage systems during the twentieth century did tropical diseases subside. As late as 1920, though, the death rate from malaria in Mississippi was 38.2 per 100,000 persons, the eighth leading cause of death in the state.[5]

For the greater part of the nineteenth century, the Mississippi Delta was as thick with canebrakes and cypress as it was with mosquitoes and malaria. But during the 1870s and 1880s, the introduction of rail lines transformed the region from an overgrown, disease-ridden swamp into an agricultural boom town with one of the fastest growth rates in the American South. Farmers flocked to the delta to exploit its central redeeming quality: a never-before-cultivated soil, capable of growing cotton so high that it could reach the height of "a man on horseback," and so thick that "a laborer could pick five hundred pounds in a single day." The transformation of the delta was particularly beneficial to blacks. Because the region was so undeveloped and labor was so scarce, employers were forced to disregard their

prejudices, and blacks were able to get jobs and wages usually reserved for whites. Visitors saw blacks working as managers, police
officers, and engineers, and they saw black laborers "making more
money than white farmers elsewhere." For a short time, there were
more black landowners in the delta than there were white.[6]

Incorporated in 1886, the town of Shaw was but one manifestation of
the wave of black in-migration to the delta. As such, Shaw began as
an agricultural community with a large black population, and it has
retained these characteristics over time. As late as 1970, 70 percent of
Shaw's 2,513 residents were black, and most of them continued to
work in agriculture or agriculture-related industries, particularly, rice,
cotton, and soybeans. Shaw experienced rapid growth initially; before
1920, its population doubled once every 10 years. But after 1920, things
started to change. Population growth stagnated between 1940 and
1960, and began a slow decline during the later part of the century.[7] A
recent study attributes the decline of Shaw and that of the broader
delta region to an economic and political system dominated by a small
and powerful white minority who used their power to enrich themselves at the expense of the poor (black) majority in the region. The de-
mise of the region was also hastened by World War I, which opened
up well-paying factory jobs in the urban North to poor delta blacks
who had previously been denied such opportunities.[8]

By the time a federal court handed down *Shaw*, the town was a very
poor place, even by the standards of Mississippi, then the poorest
state in the Union. In 1970, median family income in Shaw was
$3,268, roughly half the median family income for the state as a whole
($6,071). Twenty-four percent of the town's male labor force was un-
employed, which was six times the unemployment rate for the state as
a whole (4 percent). Fifty-three percent of the town's families lived below the poverty line, which was almost twice the poverty rate for the
state as a whole (28.9 percent). Twenty-five percent of all families in
Shaw relied on some form of public assistance, which was more than
twice the rate for the state as a whole (11 percent). For persons over age
25, the median for years of schooling was eight; for the state as a whole
it was eleven.[9]

Shaw was so poor that it did not have a public water system until
the 1930s, did not begin paving its roads until 1960, did not have sanitary sewers until 1963, and had no system for surface water drainage as late as 1970. Asked to describe how one black neighborhood

drained excess surface water, a local official offered the following testimony during the trial of *Hawkins v. Shaw*:

> Within the last week someone has come along and cleared a ditch in one section of Canaan Street. The ditch is in the shape of a spade; that is, it's one shovel wide and one shovel deep and whatever was in what is now the ditch is now heaped in a pile along the side.[10]

Because of the town's low elevation, its proximity to the Mississippi River, and high levels of rainfall, the slow development of sanitary and storm sewers had serious implications for public health. Without sanitary sewers, most households disposed of their sewage in open ditches that extended into nearby bayous. When the bayous reached capacity, overflowing sewage tainted nearby surface wells, spreading typhoid, dysentery, and other diarrheal diseases. In addition, without storm sewers, excess water often lay stagnant, a breeding ground for mosquitoes carrying malaria and yellow fever.[11]

Lessons from the History of Shaw

Three lessons can be drawn from the history of Shaw. First, the town's economic and political development make it an outlier, particularly with regard to its extreme poverty and its late installation of water and sewer systems. While Shaw first installed a water system during the 1930s, and its sewer system in the 1960s, all major American cities began installing their water and sewer systems before 1900. (The extent to which other American cities developed their water and sewer systems is documented in chapter 3.) Second, the patterns of segregation observed in Shaw facilitated efforts to discriminate in the provision of water and sewer systems, as well as other municipal services. In a more integrated town it would have been difficult to adversely serve blacks without also adversely serving whites, given the networked structure of water and sewer mains. In this way, Shaw's failure to provide adequate sanitary services to black neighborhoods was a historical anomaly. If Shaw had built its water and sewer systems during the nineteenth century when towns and cities were more integrated, as all major American cities had done, town officials would have had a much harder time denying blacks water and sewer service because it would have also required them to deny service to whites.

Third, although a federal appeals court rejected claims made by the town that legitimate policy concerns might have helped generate racial

disparities in access to various municipal services, a geographic overview of the town suggests the courts might have been in error. The
racial geography of Shaw was such that whites lived in the densely
populated center of town, while African Americans lived in the less
densely populated periphery. Because whites lived in areas with relatively high population densities and areas with high population density required larger water mains than areas with low densities, it comes
as no surprise that black homes would have been served by smaller
water mains than white homes. By the same token, the lag in bringing sewer service to African-American households might have been
caused by the fact that it took longer to lay mains and bring service
to peripheral areas with low population densities. Recall that Shaw
did not even begin building a sanitary sewer system, for either whites
or blacks, until 1963. While this does not exonerate town officials of
wrongdoing, it does corroborate the view that *Shaw* was a decision of
little practical importance for more typical American cities and towns.

Assessing the Legal Significance of Hawkins v. Shaw

To assess the legal significance of *Hawkins v. Shaw*, table 5.1 lists the
number of times subsequent court decisions have cited this decision as
well as other civil rights-related decisions. It is clear from this table that
despite initial predictions, *Shaw* has proven to be nowhere near as
important as *Brown*. Citations to *Brown* exceed citations to *Shaw* by a
factor of 37. One might (correctly) argue that few cases in American
history are as significant as *Brown*, and so this case is probably an unrealistic benchmark. *Shaw*, though, has not been cited as often as *Bakke*,
or even lesser-known cases such as *Green v. County Board of New Kent
County* and *Swann v. Charlotte-Mecklenburg Board of Education*.

Cases with citation counts similar to *Shaw*'s include *Watson v. Memphis* and *Gilmore v. Montgomery*. In *Watson*, black residents of Memphis
sued to require the city to desegregate public parks, pools, and other
public recreational facilities in a timely manner. In *Gilmore*, black residents of Montgomery, Alabama, sued to stop a policy that allowed
private schools with race-based admissions policies (i.e., schools that
excluded blacks) to use public pools and other publicly owned struc-
tures. *Gilmore* appears to have been a natural and logical extension of
Norwood v. Harris, a decision that forced Mississippi to stop loaning
state-owned textbooks to children attending racially segregated private
schools (see table 5.1).

Table 5.1
Major Civil Rights Cases: Some Citation Counts

Case	Substantive issue	No. of citations
Brown v. Board of Education	Racially segregated schools in Topeka, Kansas	9,078
University of California v. Bakke	Affirmative action in college admissions	3,333
Norwood v. Harris	State-owned textbooks loaned to children attending racially segregated private schools	425
Gilmore v. Montgomery	Private schools with race-based admissions policies used public pools, buildings, etc.	208
Green v. New Kent County	Parents chose the public school their child attended and kept schools segregated by race	1,431
Swann v. Charlotte	Busing school children in North Carolina to achieve racially integrated public schools	1,919
Watson v. Memphis	Segregated public parks, pools, and other recreational facilities in Memphis, Tennessee	244
Hawkins v. Shaw	See text	241
Washington v. Davis	Racial bias in verbal test administered to police recruits in Washington, D.C.	3,943

Sources: Lexis/Nexis (accessed through Academic Universe) and court reporters cited in table.
Note: The exact citation for each case is as follows in order of appearance in the table: *Brown*, 347 U.S. 483 (1954) and 349 U.S. 294 (1955); *Bakke* 438 U.S. 265 (1979); *Norwood* 413 U.S. 455 (1973); *Gilmore* 417 U.S. 556 (1974); *Green* 391 U.S. 430 (1968); *Swann* 402 U.S. 1 (1971); *Watson* 373 U.S. 526 (1963); *Hawkins* 437 F.2d 1286 (1970) and 461 F.2d 1171 (1972); *Washington* 426 U.S. 229 (1976).

One concern with using citations to assess the legal significance of a particular court decision is that citations alone tell us almost nothing about the effect of that decision on the actual implementation of public policy. To see this, imagine a world where all laws are enforced immediately and costlessly. In such a world, all the courts need to do is establish a legal rule once, and all subsequent actors will obey that rule forever. And in such a world, it is possible that although the *Shaw* decision has not been cited frequently, it has lead to substantial changes in the provision of water and sewer facilities and greatly increased access to these facilities for African Americans.

The problems with this line of thought are twofold. First, one wonders why public water and sewer services would have been so different from public schooling. More precisely, in the case of education funding and desegregation, there is no evidence that local school boards and universities desegregated immediately following *Brown v. Board of Education*. On the contrary, thousands of additional legal battles had to be fought before local school boards conceded that *Brown* applied to their set of ostensibly peculiar circumstances. Second, evidence presented later in this chapter shows that 10 years *before* the Shaw decision was handed down, there were no meaningful differences in the rate at which blacks and whites were connected to public water and sewer lines. This evidence is based on a sample of roughly 250,000 households taken from the U.S. Census. One might argue that cities equalized access to water and sewer lines in anticipation of *Shaw*, but again, if this is correct, one wonders why local school boards did not desegregate in anticipation of *Brown*.

A more realistic objection to the use of citation counts is that legal decisions are important, not merely because the rules they establish affect the particular policy being litigated, but also because the rules they establish can affect a much broader set of policies. In this way, it is important to be clear on exactly what the 241 cases that cited *Shaw* were, and were not, about. Most were not about discrimination in the provision of public water and sewer services. As the next section shows, only six other municipalities in the United States have been found guilty of discriminating in the provision of these services.

Most of the decisions that have cited *Shaw* do so because of the evidentiary standard it articulated regarding the existence of discrimination. In particular, in *Shaw*, the courts ruled that "in order to prevail in a case of this type it is *not* necessary to prove intent, motive, or purpose to discriminate on the part of city officials" [emphasis added].[12] The outcome spoke for itself: African-American households were connected to public sewers at much lower rates than whites and whatever the intent, that outcome was inconsistent with a constitution that guaranteed equal protection under the law. This evidentiary standard, not the specific application of the Fourteenth Amendment protections to public water and sewer systems, is what gives *Shaw* whatever legal significance it has. Moreover, this legal significance has declined over time because the evidentiary standard it applied has been overturned in recent years by *Washington v. Davis*. In *Washington*, the U.S. Supreme Court ruled that racial disparities in outcomes (in this case in verbal tests administered to police department recruits) do not by themselves prove that a group has been discriminated against. Citations to *Washington* exceed citations to *Shaw* by a factor of 16 (see table 5.1).[13]

Other Cities That Have Been Sued

Apart from Shaw, six municipalities in the United States have been found guilty of discriminating in the provision of public water and sewer services: Apopka, Arcadia, Dade City, Delray Beach, and Fort Myers, all in Florida; and Lackawanna, New York. Like Shaw, these towns were all sued during the 1970s and early 1980s, following the Civil Rights movement. It is notable that as in Shaw, none of the litigation in these cases reached the U.S. Supreme Court. All of the cases were decided by a federal appeals court or a district court.

The suits brought against Apopka, Arcadia, and Fort Myers revolved around the same set of issues as those raised in the suit against Shaw. The municipalities in question had failed to install water and sewer mains in black residential areas, or, in the case of Arcadia, had installed water mains that were too small and therefore did not provide adequate water pressure. In the other three cases there is not a direct parallel with *Shaw*. Specifically, the suit brought against Dade City differs from *Shaw* in that the plaintiffs made no claims that water and sanitary sewer service in the town's black residential area was inadequate; the suit sought only to rectify inequities in storm water drainage. The suits brought against Delray Beach and Lackawanna differ from Shaw in that the plaintiffs made no claims that the cities involved had provided inadequate access to public water and sewer lines in existing black residential areas. Rather, the plaintiffs sought relief because Delray and Lackawanna had refused to offer water and sewer service to planned low-income housing complexes. The cities had denied these services in an effort to forestall construction of the complexes. These contrasts suggest that there have been only three cases that involved the same basic issues as those raised by *Shaw*.

Table 5.2 lists the six municipalities that have been successfully sued and their characteristics, along with those of Shaw. Like Shaw, all of the towns were small; no town had a population greater than 30,000 in 1960 and three had a population of less than 4,500. As for the development of their water and sewer systems, all of the towns reported in table 5.2 were like Shaw in that they lagged far behind the larger cities described in chapter 3. Excluding Shaw, two of the six towns had no

Table 5.2
Cities Sued for Discriminating in the Provision of Public Water and Sewer Services

Town	Year of suit	Population, 1960		Water system, 1915		Sewer system, 1922	
		Total	% Black	Built	% Connected	Built	% Connected
Apopka, Fla.	1983	3,578	0.298	After 1915	0.00	After 1922	0.00
Arcadia, Fla.	1978	5,889	0.365	1907	0.60	1907	0.50
Dade City, Fla.	1984	4,241	0.293	1914	0.75	1915	0.30
Delray Beach, Fla.	1974	12,230	0.439	1914	0.33	After 1922	0.00
Fort Myers, Fla.	1980	22,523	0.258	1911	0.50	1911	0.50
Lackawanna, N.Y.	1970	29,564	0.051	?	?	?	?
Shaw, Miss.	1969–1972	2,062	0.644	After 1915	0.00	1963	0.00

Sources: *Dowdell et al. v. Apopka*, 698 F.2d 1181 (1983); *Ammons, Dobson et al. v. Dade City*, 594 F. Supp. 1274 (1984); *Johnson v. City of Arcadia*, 450 F. Supp. 1363 (1978); *Kennedy Park Homes Association v. City of Lackawanna*, 436 F.2d 108 (1970); *United Farmworkers of Florida Housing Project, Inc. v. City of Delray Beach*, 493 F.2d 799 (1974); *Hawkins v. Town of Shaw*, 461 F.2d 1171 (1972); *Harris v. City of Fort Myers*, 624 F.2d 1321 (1980). Data on population in 1960 come from the 1960 census. Data on water systems for towns in Florida come from the Florida State Board of Health, *Biennial Reports*, 1914–1915 and 1921–1922.

water system at all by 1915, and three of them had no sewer system by 1922. In no town did the sewer system extend to more than half the population, and in most towns the water system did not reach more than half the population. Recall from chapter 3 that in 1915 cities that ranked at the bottom 5 percent in terms of the development of their water systems had at least 67 percent of their populations connected, and that in 1909 cities that ranked in the bottom 5 percent in terms of the development of their sewer systems had at least 26 percent of their populations connected (see table 3.1).

The towns reported in table 5.2 were like Shaw in one additional and important respect. They were extremely segregated, with blacks limited to a particular geographic area of the town. In this way Shaw and these other municipalities were different from major American cities *at the turn of the century*, where and when black households were spread throughout the city in question (see chapters 3 and 4). For example, when a federal court found Apopka guilty of discrimination, the court described how a segregation ordinance in effect until 1968 forced local blacks to live on the south side of the railroad tracks running through the town. According to the court, this ordinance "contributed to the ghetto-like qualities of the [single] black residential area."[14] Similarly, a district court described how 90 percent of all African Americans in Dade City lived in a single residential area defined by two sets of railroad tracks and a major thoroughfare. According to the court, this area "formed almost a perfect triangle in the southeastern region of the city."[15] And again in *Johnson et al. v. Arcadia*, a federal court wrote:

The City of Arcadia has developed according to a strict pattern of residential racial segregation. The entire black community is bordered by railroad tracks to the east, north, and west.... No blacks reside anywhere outside this small geographical area in the southwest portion of Arcadia.[16]

Finally, in *Kennedy Park Homes Association v. City of Lackawanna*, another federal court offered the following description of racial segregation and isolation in Lackawanna:

We have a three-ward city with 98.9 percent of all of its nonwhite citizens living in the First Ward. The Second Ward ... has only one nonwhite person, while only 29 nonwhites reside in the Third Ward. The Bethlehem Steel Company's plant, with its more than 20,000 employees, occupies at least half the land area of the First Ward.... To add insult to injury, a series of parallel railroad tracks serves the steel mill, running along the east boundary of the First Ward and physically separating it from the rest of the City. Indeed the only traffic connection between the two is a single bridge that spans the railroad tracks at Ridge Road.[17]

The import of all this is clear; like Shaw, the other municipalities that have been successfully sued for discriminating in the provision of water and sewer services differed from most American cities and towns in two important respects. First, they had built their systems late in the twentieth century and second, they were extremely segregated, so that black households were located almost exclusively in one part of town and were therefore easily denied service. These patterns bolster the argument developed in chapters 3 and 4 that residential segregation facilitated efforts to deny African-American households access to public water and sewer lines. There are two cases, those that involve Delray Beach and Lackawanna, that do not fit this particular construct, but nonetheless, they do not contradict the argument that segregation mattered. As stated earlier, these cases involved local governments that had refused to extend water and sewer lines to planned low-income housing complexes in an effort to forestall their construction.

At this point it is useful to describe one other way that Shaw, Apopka, Arcadia, etc., differed from other cities and towns. By the late twentieth century, many cities and towns in the United States provided sewers and other public services based solely on neighborhood demand and the willingness of concerned homeowners to pay for those services. In contrast, the town of Shaw did not follow such procedures and claimed to provide services to all who requested them, without charging special fees. Consider the case of Prattville, Alabama, another tiny southern town that was sued for failing to provide black neighborhoods with water and sewer lines. In Prattville, neighborhoods received water and sewer lines when 51 percent of the residents petitioned the local government to have such lines installed. Once the local government had been petitioned, homeowners in the neighborhood had their property values reassessed so that their taxes rose, and the water and sewer lines were installed. There was no evidence that local officials in Prattville had refused to respond to the petitioning of black households; there was only evidence that black neighborhoods had never filed the necessary petitions and had never paid the associated tax assessments. In this case, the courts found Prattville innocent of the charges that it had discriminated in the distribution of public water and sewer services, although there was evidence the city had discriminated in the provision of park areas for black residents. When municipalities financed public water and sewer lines in the same way Prattville had—and this mode of financing appears to have grown increasingly common over time—it becomes difficult to sustain the idea that public officials discriminated.[18]

5.3 Evidence of Equal Access to Public Water and Sewer Facilities in 1960

The argument I have advanced thus far is that Shaw represents an exception that proves a more general rule. It is rare for cities and towns in the United States to be successfully sued for failing to provide adequate water and sewer services to African-American households. There is a simple reason for this. Discriminating in the provision of public water is costly because it increases the risk of epidemic diseases and because, given the networked structure of water and sewer systems, it is difficult to deny black households service without also denying service to white households.

If this argument is correct, we should observe racial parity in access to public water and sewer lines in the years preceding the *Shaw* decision. To test this proposition, this section employs household-level data derived from the Integrated Public Use Micro Data Series.[19] As discussed briefly in chapter 4, the IPUMS data are composed of large and random samples from various U.S. censuses. These data are well known, widely used, and require only brief explanatory comments.

For the analysis here, a large and randomly selected group of households from the 1960 census was downloaded from the IPUMS electronic data extraction system. The sample represents 1 percent of all households that responded to U.S. census takers' questions regarding the household's access to public water and sewer lines. The sample contains 262,232 household-level observations. With these data it is possible to identify differences in the rates at which white-headed households and African-American-headed households were connected to local water and sewer lines as of 1960, before the Civil Rights movement and the ruling in *Hawkins v. Shaw*. It is also possible to identify other relevant household characteristics, including such things as income, poverty status, education, marital status, and whether the household in question was located in a central city, a suburb, or a nonmetropolitan area. (Unfortunately, however, the IPUMS does not report the household's specific metropolitan area, which would be useful

for the analysis here.) These additional characteristics allow one to disentangle the effects of race from income, poverty, education, marital
status, and the like.

Before turning to the analysis, it is important to note that census data
will understate the true level of accessibility to public water and sewer
lines, for both whites and blacks. This is because it was possible for a
household to front on a water or sewer main while at the same time
deciding not to connect to it. The rates at which households actually
connected to public water and sewer mains could be much lower than
the rates at which they fronted those mains. In chapter 4 I used data on
frontage rates from turn-of-the-century cities and arrived at conclusions very similar to those reported here. Hence the analysis in this
chapter is best thought of as complementing rather than superseding
or overturning the previous analysis.

Data and Some Preliminary Findings

If cities and towns in the United States systematically denied African-
American households access to public water and sewer lines in the pre-
Shaw era, one would expect to observe large disparities in the rates at
which blacks and whites were connected to these facilities in 1960.
Based on the IPUMS sample, table 5.3 presents some descriptive statistics on this question. These data reveal that there were interracial disparities in connection rates, although the patterns that emerge do not
really support the idea that cities systematically discriminated against
blacks in these services. In the non-South, black households were actually 3 percentage points more likely than white households to have
had access to public water facilities and 5 points more likely to have
sewer hookups; while in the South, black households were 7 percentage points less likely than white households to have had public water
and 9 points less likely to be connected to a sewer line. Although these
black-white differences are statistically significant, they are quite small
relative to differences in other racial groups. For example, Chinese
households in the North were 25 percentage points more likely than
white households to have had public water and Japanese households
were 11 points more likely. Clearly it would be a mistake to infer from
these differences that municipal authorities in the North gave preference to African-American, Chinese, and Japanese households over
white households when they installed water and sewer mains.

Table 5.3
Race and Connections to Public Water and Sewer Lines in the United States, 1960

Race of household head	No. of households		Proportion of households connected to			
			Public water		Public sewer	
	North	South	North	South	North	South
Black	3,587	12,683	0.726	0.468	0.580	0.275
White	187,685	56,744	0.697	0.596	0.534	0.394
American Indian	642	92	0.382	0.163	0.246	0.098
Chinese	91	8	0.945	1.000	0.703	0.625
Japanese	310	7	0.806	0.714	0.442	0.571
Other Asian	223	3	0.834	0.667	0.444	0.667
Other nonwhite	155	2	0.735	0.500	0.329	0.500
Regional subtotal (average)	192,693	69,531	(0.697)	(0.572)	(0.534)	(0.372)
Total (average)	262,232		(0.664)		(0.491)	

Source: Ruggles and Sobek, *Integrated Public Use Micro Data Series* (hereafter cited as IPUMS).

The interracial disparities reported in table 5.3 might stem from any number of causes. For example, individuals located in the central part of cities, which had complete water and sewer systems as early as 1900, would have been much more likely to have had service, regardless of their race, than individuals located in suburban areas or in other nonmetropolitan areas, which had lower population densities and were only recently settled. As of 1960, black households in the non-South were 2.2 times more likely than white households to have resided in the central part of cities. In the South, the differential between the rates at which black and white households located in city centers was about one-third the size of the differential in the North. Other possible and benign explanations might include interracial differences in demand for public water and sewer connections stemming from such things as income, education, poverty status, and labor market status. African-American households were disadvantaged in most of these categories. In the full 1960 IPUMS sample, black households were 2.5 times more likely than white households to have been in poverty, and were 2 times more likely than white households to have had a household head who was unemployed.

Table 5.4 addresses concerns surrounding the location of black and white households. More precisely, this table presents statistics on access to public water and sewer lines according to the location of households, whether in the central part of cities, the suburbs, or outside standard metropolitan areas. This table excludes households for which it was not possible to identify locations precisely. For example, for some households located in metropolitan areas it is not possible to identify their location in relation to the city center. (See table 5.5 for a more complete description of the variables characterizing a household's metropolitan status.) Several notable patterns emerge from table 5.4. Regardless of their race, households located outside metropolitan areas have the lowest connection rates to public water and sewer lines. Households located in suburbs have higher connection rates, and households located in the central part of cities have the highest connection rates. In central city areas, differences between black and white connection rates are very small, and overall connection rates are usually above 95 percent. The large differences in black and white connection rates appear only outside the central part of cities, in suburbs and nonmetropolitan areas. It is interesting to note that Chinese and Japanese households tend to have much higher connection rates to public water and sewer lines than either black or white households.

Table 5.4
Race, Location, and Connections to Public Water and Sewer Lines

	Black			White			Chinese			Japanese		
	No. of house- holds	% Con- nected to water	% Con- nected to sewer	No. of house- holds	% Con- nected to water	% Con- nected to sewer	No. of house- holds	% Con- nected to water	% Con- nected to sewer	No. of house- holds	% Con- nected to water	% Con- nected to sewer
Full sample												
Not in metro area	9,145	0.515	0.346	99,071	0.649	0.510	26	0.923	0.885	39	0.615	0.487
In metro area												
Central city	412	0.942	0.837	4,017	0.972	0.881	...	...	...	...	...	...
Not in central city (suburb)	3,004	0.679	0.430	87,086	0.788	0.555	40	1.00	0.700	80	0.624	0.529
South												
Not in metro area	7,873	0.481	0.307	33,984	0.562	0.409	...	...	...	...	...	...
In metro area												
Central city	309	0.932	0.796	1,501	0.958	0.848	...	...	...	...	...	...
Not in central city (suburb)	1,543	0.581	0.229	13,098	0.751	0.404	6	1.00	0.667	3	0.667	0.333
Non-South												
Not in metro area	1,272	0.725	0.593	65,087	0.694	0.562	26	0.917	0.917	39	0.622	0.486
In metro area												
Central city	103	0.971	0.961	2,516	0.980	0.901	...	...	...	...	...	...
Not in central city (suburb)	1,461	0.783	0.643	73,988	0.794	0.582	34	1.00	0.706	77	0.622	0.537

Source: IPUMS.
Note: ..., no observations.

Table 5.5
List of Control Variables

Short definition	Full description
Race ($\mathbf{X}_1$)	A series of dummy variables indicating race: African American, American Indian, Chinese, Japanese, other Asian, other non white race, and white (omitted category).
Metropolitan status ($\mathbf{X}_2$)	A series of dummy variables indicating household's location: central city; metro area, not central city; central city status unknown; outside metro area; and metropolitan status unknown.
Economic status ($\mathbf{X}_3$)	A continuous variable indicating total family income and a series of dummy variables indicating poverty status and labor force status of household head (employed, unemployed, or not actively seeking employment).
Demographic status ($\mathbf{X}_4$)	A continuous variable indicating age and a series of dummy variables indicating the household head's marital status (married, single, divorced, or separated), number of children in home, and sex of household head.
Housing stock ($\mathbf{X}_5$)	A series of dummy variables indicating whether the structure was owned or rented, a mobile home, had a basement, units in structure, and year built.
State dummies ($\boldsymbol{a}_0$)	A series of dummy variables indicating household's state of residence.

Source: See text.

Estimating Strategy

To control for location and other contingencies more formally, data on a variety of household characteristics other than race were collected and probit models of the following form estimated:

$$\text{prob}(y_i = 1) = \Phi(\boldsymbol{a}_0 + \mathbf{X}_{1i}\beta_1 + \mathbf{X}_{2i}\beta_2 + \mathbf{X}_{3i}\beta_3 + \mathbf{X}_{4i}\beta_4 + \mathbf{X}_{5i}\beta_5), \qquad (5.1)$$

where y_i equals one if household i was connected to public water (sewer) and zero otherwise; Φ is the cumulative normal distribution; $\boldsymbol{a}_0$ is a vector of fifty dummy variables indicating the state of residence for a household i; $\mathbf{X}_{1i}$ is a vector of dummy variables indicating the race of the household head; $\mathbf{X}_{2i}$ is a vector of dummy variables indicating whether the household lived in the central city, a suburb, or a nonmetropolitan area; $\mathbf{X}_{3i}$ is a vector of variables describing the household's economic status (e.g., poverty status, income, and employment); $\mathbf{X}_{4i}$ is a vector of variables describing the household's demographic status (e.g., whether the head of household was married, age of household head, and number of children in home); and X_{5i} is a vector of dummy variables indicating the structural characteristics of the household's dwelling (e.g., age of structure, number of units in structure, mobile home, and whether the unit was owned or rented). Table 5.5 provides a more complete description of the control variables used.

Before turning to the results, two caveats about this regression approach need to be stated. First, there is no reasonable way in this procedure to control for the possibility that blacks and/or whites self-selected areas without public water or sewer lines. Obviously homes in areas without public water and sewer services were much less expensive than those with these services, and to the extent that blacks were poorer than whites, they might have chosen to live in such areas deliberately, independent of any choice by public authorities to discriminate. Including variables such as income and labor force status controls for some of these issues, but they can never capture all of the unobserved heterogeneity across the races. As a result, the regression results reported here probably overstate the extent of discrimination on the part of public providers of water and sewer services. Second, the actual regressions estimated vary in the precision in which they control for locational differences across the races. Specifically, some regressions include state dummies; others include state-specific metropolitan dummies, meaning that state dummies have been interacted with the metropolitan status dummies; and some regressions include neither the state dummies nor the state-metro interaction dummies.

Regression Results

Table 5.6 contains the regression results on connection rates to public water systems for the sample and for households located in the South and non-South. Note that the table gives the estimated change in probability resulting from a 0/1 change in the black dummy. The estimate of primary interest is the effect of race on the probability of a household having been connected to public water in 1960. In the full sample, black households are no less likely than white ones to have been connected to public water supplies. The estimated change in probability is tiny, statistically and substantively, and this finding is robust to the inclusion or exclusion of state dummies and state-specific metro dummies (see regressions 1a, 1b, and 1c). The same is true if the sample

Table 5.6
Race and Access to Public Water: Regression Results

	Full sample			South only			non-South only		
	1a	1b	1c	2a	2b	2c	3a	3b	3c
=1 if public water	Dependent variable			Dependent variable			Dependent variable		
=1 if black household	−0.008	0.002	−0.002	−0.016	−0.007	−0.007	0.046	0.027	0.025
	(0.004)	(0.004)	(0.004)	(0.006)	(0.006)	(0.006)	(0.007)	(0.008)	(0.008)
Other race	Yes	Yes	Yes	Yes	Yes	Yes	Yes	Yes	Yes
Metro. status	Yes	Yes	Yes	Yes	Yes	Yes	Yes	Yes	Yes
Economic status	Yes	Yes	Yes	Yes	Yes	Yes	Yes	Yes	Yes
Demographic status	Yes	Yes	Yes	Yes	Yes	Yes	Yes	Yes	Yes
Housing	Yes	Yes	Yes	Yes	Yes	Yes	Yes	Yes	Yes
State	No	Yes	No	No	Yes	No	No	Yes	No
State/Metro	No	No	Yes	No	No	Yes	No	No	Yes
No. of observations	262,232	262,232	261,972	69,531	69,531	69,531	192,693	192,693	192,433
Prob. $> \chi^2$	0.000	0.000	0.000	0.000	0.000	0.000	0.000	0.000	0.000
Pseudo R^2	0.140	0.197	0.232	0.138	0.188	0.192	0.135	0.193	0.239

Source: See text.
Notes: Standard errors are in parentheses. Also, this table reports the estimated change in probability resulting from a 0/1 change in the black dummy.

Table 5.7
Race and Access to Public Sewers: Regression Results

	Full sample			South only			non-South only		
	1a	1b	1c	2a	2b	2c	3a	3b	3c
	Dependent variable			Dependent variable			Dependent variable		
=1 if public sewer									
=1 if black household	−0.044	−0.021	−0.030	−0.027	−0.029	−0.029	0.061	0.032	0.029
	(0.005)	(0.005)	(0.005)	(0.005)	(0.006)	(0.006)	(0.009)	(0.009)	(0.010)
Other race	Yes	Yes	Yes	Yes	Yes	Yes	Yes	Yes	Yes
Metro. status	Yes	Yes	Yes	Yes	Yes	Yes	Yes	Yes	Yes
Economic status	Yes	Yes	Yes	Yes	Yes	Yes	Yes	Yes	Yes
Demographic status	Yes	Yes	Yes	Yes	Yes	Yes	Yes	Yes	Yes
Housing	Yes	Yes	Yes	Yes	Yes	Yes	Yes	Yes	Yes
State	No	Yes	No	No	Yes	No	No	Yes	No
State/Metro	No	No	Yes	No	No	Yes	No	No	Yes
No. of observations	262,232	262,232	261,925	69,539	69,539	69,539	192,693	192,693	192,386
Prob. $> \chi^2$	0.000	0.000	0.000	0.000	0.000	0.000	0.000	0.000	0.000
Pseudo R^2	0.121	0.185	0.218	0.124	0.180	0.187	0.113	0.173	0.214

Source: See text.
Notes: Standard errors are in parentheses. Also, this table reports the estimated change in probability resulting from a 0/1 change in the black dummy.

is restricted exclusively to households located in the South. Again, the black households are no less likely than white ones to have had public water (see regressions 2a, 2b, and 2c). In the non-South, after controlling for all other factors, black households are a few percentage points more likely than white ones to have been connected to public water lines (see regressions 3a, 3b, and 3c).

Table 5.7 reports the results for public sewers. In the full sample, black households are 2 to 4 percentage points (3 percent) less likely than white households to have been connected to public sewers (see regressions 1a, 1b, and 1c). In the South, there is stronger evidence of discrimination, and black households are about 3 percentage points (8 percent) less likely than white households to have been connected to public sewers (see regressions 2a, 2b, and 2c). In the non-South, black households appear 3 to 6 percentage points (6 to 11 percent) more likely than white households to have been connected to public sewers.

5.4 Conclusions

This chapter has explored the central paradox of *Shaw*: How is it that a legal decision that promised so much in the way of future litigation and social improvement, a decision heralded as the next *Brown v. Board of Education* no less, amounted to so little? The argument developed here suggests that most cities and towns in America have avoided lawsuits like *Hawkins v. Shaw* because before the Civil Rights movement ever began, they were already providing black families with about the same level of water and sewer services as similarly situated white families. Besides the evidence presented elsewhere in this book, the history of Shaw supports this proposition. It is clear that in 1960 this town had more in common with the third world than it did with a developed country. Shaw was not like most American towns and it is not surprising that such a place would produce a legal situation and ruling that would prove to have little relevance for the typical American city.

Overall, the patterns identified in this chapter suggest that racial disparities in connection rates to local water and sewer systems do not necessarily imply that local authorities were discriminating in the provision of these services, unless one wants to argue that local governments gave preference to Chinese and Japanese households over white households in extending public water and sewer lines. The statistical findings here leave no doubt. Holding everything else constant, there were only trivial differences in the rates at which black and white households connected to public water and sewer lines. Shaw and the handful of other cities that have been found guilty of discrimination in this area are outliers, with little relationship to most American cities and towns.

6   Water Filtration: Who Benefitted and Why

6.1   An Introduction

The econometric tests in this chapter build on the following intuition: If blacks generally did not have access to public water systems, or had relatively limited access, improvements in water quality would have benefitted whites disproportionately. In such a world, the installation of water filters would have reduced white waterborne disease rates, but had little effect on black disease rates. Later in the chapter I test this proposition using formal regression models, but first, I describe the data that are used in that estimation and present some cruder, preliminary analyses of the data. The preliminary analyses and discussion serve two purposes. First, those readers who are unaccustomed to econometric approaches will find the less formal preliminary analyses more accessible. Second, these analyses will help explain the empirical work that follows.

6.2   The Data and Some Preliminary Findings

To analyze the relationships between disease and water quality across racial groups, a panel of thirty-three cities was assembled. For each city in the panel there are annual data on typhoid rates by race and information on when, if ever, the city installed a water filter or chlorination system. Typhoid rates are measured as deaths from typhoid per 100,000 persons. Table 6.1 lists the cities included in the panel and the years they were observed. The cities span the United States, including places in the North and South and the East and West. The panel is unbalanced. Most cities were observed from 1906 through 1920, but three cities—Charleston, South Carolina; Charlotte, North Carolina; and Pittsburgh, Pennsylvania—were observed for much longer periods.

118

Chapter 6

Table 6.1
Cities Included in Analysis of Panel Data

City and state	Years observed
Atlanta, Ga.*	1906–1920
Augusta, Ga.*	1913–1920
Baltimore, Md.*	1906–1920
Birmingham, Ala.*	1908–1920
Boston, Mass.*	1908–1920
Charleston, SC.*	1890–1920
Charlotte, NC.	1890–1919
Chicago, Ill.	1908–1920
Cincinnati, Ohio	1908–1920
Columbus, Ohio	1910–1920
Covington, Ky.*	1911–1919
Jacksonville, Fla.	1906–1920
Kansas City, Kan.	1908–1920
Kansas City, Mo.	1906–1920
Los Angeles, Calif.	1910–1920
Louisville, Ky.	1906–1920
Lynchburg, Va.	1906–1920
Memphis, Tenn.*	1906–1920
Montgomery, Ala.	1908–1920
Nashville, Tenn.	1906–1920
New Orleans, La.	1906–1920
Newport, Ky.	1911–1919
New York, NY.	1910–1920
Norfolk, Va.*	1906–1920
Philadelphia, Pa.	1908–1920
Pittsburgh, Pa.	1888–1920
Richmond, Va.	1906–1920
St. Louis, Mo.	1908–1920
San Antonio, Texas*	1906–1920
San Francisco, Calif.*	1909–1920
Savannah, Ga.*	1906–1920
Washington, D.C.	1906–1920
Wilmington, Del.	1906–1920

Sources: Data on typhoid rates are from Bureau of Census, *Mortality Statistics* and various state and local public health departments. Data on water filtration come from the *McGraw Directory of American Water Companies* (no author) and Bureau of Census, *General Statistics of Cities*, 1915.
Note: An asterisk indicates that the city did not install a water filter or begin chlorinating its water during the period for which it is observed.

Table 6.2
Descriptive Statistics for Panel Data

	Full sample		Regional subsamples[b]				Segregation subsamples[c]			
			South		Non-South		Segregated		Integrated	
Variable[a]	μ	σ	μ	σ	μ	σ	μ	σ	μ	σ
y^b	41.4	37.4	48.1	33.7	35.0	39.6	33.9	27.1	44.0	40.5
y^w	28.5	26.1	39.1	29.2	18.3	17.4	25.3	22.3	26.1	21.9
$(y^b - y^w)$	12.9	27.5	8.95	27.3	16.6	27.2	8.68	18.1	18.0	27.0
$(y^b)/(y^w)$	1.77	1.37	1.49	1.05	2.02	1.58	1.61	1.04	2.07	1.62
No. of observations	484		236		248		206		190	

Source: See text.
Note: μ, mean; σ, standard deviation.
[a] y^b, black typhoid rates; y^w, white typhoid rates. Typhoid rates are measured as deaths per 100,000 persons from typhoid fever.
[b] For the list of cities included in the South and non-South samples, see the notes following tables 6.4 and 6.5.
[c] For the list of cities included in the integrated and segregated samples, see the notes following tables 6.6 and 6.7.

Table 6.1 also indicates with an asterisk the cities that did not install water filters during the period they were observed. Of the thirty-three cities, eleven did not install water purification systems.

Table 6.2 contains some descriptive statistics on typhoid death rates for the full sample of cities and for two sets of subsamples. The latter are divided by region (South, non-South) and by the level of residential segregation (segregated or integrated). The segregation subsamples are explained in greater detail later. For the moment, simply note that segregated cities are those with an above-average level of segregation, and integrated cities are those with a below-average level. (Cities for which no measures of residential segregation are available are excluded from the analysis.) In the full sample of cities, black typhoid death rates are 45 percent greater than those for whites. There is, however, variation in the disparities in interracial disease across regions. In the North, black typhoid death rates are nearly twice white rates; in the South, black rates are only 23 percent greater than those for whites.[1]

To explore the effects of water filtration on deaths from diseases, figures 6.1 and 6.2 plot average typhoid death rates by race from 1910 to 1920 in cities that installed filters and in those that did not. In the average city, after filters were installed, black typhoid death rates fell

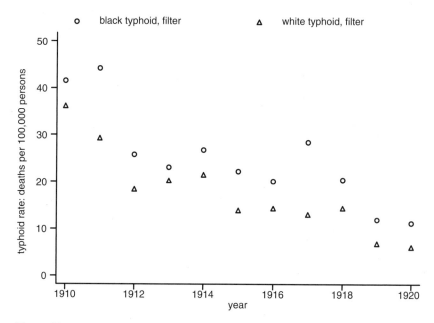

Figure 6.1
Average black and white typhoid death rates in cities with water filters. Source: See text.

from about 40 per 100,000 persons in 1910 to 8 in 1920; in the same period, white rates fell from 35 to 6 deaths per 100,000 persons (see figure 6.1). In the average city that did not install filters, there were also reductions in typhoid death rates, although they were less dramatic; black rates fell from about 50 to 20 per 100,000 persons and white rates fell from 30 to 10 deaths per 100,000 persons (see figure 6.2). These figures suggest that there was more absolute improvement in black and white typhoid death rates in cities that installed filters than in those that did not. In other words, blacks benefitted from improvements in water quality, challenging the idea that all black households were excluded from public water systems. Combined, figures 6.1 and 6.2 seem to make a powerful case for using city-specific time trends in attempting to isolate the effects of water filtration. The fact that typhoid death rates were falling in cities that did not install filters suggests that typhoid rates would have fallen in the filtering cities, even in the absence of any improvements those cities made in water purification. On the other hand, as explained in chapter 7, including city-specific trends might generate biased estimates if the effects of short-term oscillations overwhelm longer-term secular trends.

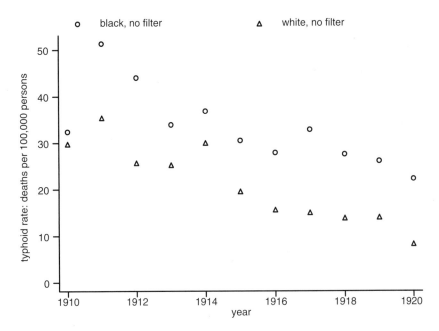

Figure 6.2
Average black and white typhoid death rates in cities without water filters. Source: See text.

To explore the effects of water filtration on interracial disparities in disease rates, figures 6.3 and 6.4 plot the difference between average black and white typhoid death rates, and the ratio of these rates in cities that installed filters and in those that did not. The data series extend from 1910 to 1920. As figure 6.3 shows, the difference between black and white typhoid death rates in cities that did not install filters was, on average, higher than the difference in cities that did install filters. Also, while there are no discernible trends before 1915, after 1915 it appears that the difference in black and white typhoid rates in non-filtering cities rose, while the difference in filtering cities remained constant. As figure 6.4 shows, the ratio of average black to white typhoid death rates remained constant in filtering cities, while it rose sharply after 1915 in nonfiltering cities. The patterns in figures 6.3 and 6.4 suggest that water filtration and purification did not benefit whites disproportionately. They also suggest that in the absence of improvements in water quality, black disease rates would have worsened, at least relative to those for whites. The results contradict the hypothesis that all black households were excluded from public water systems.

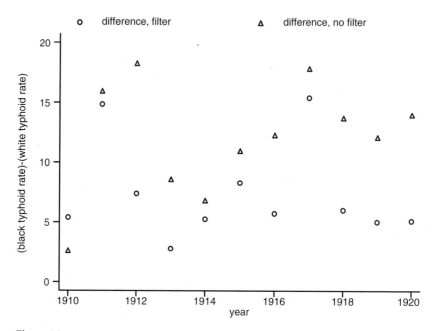

Figure 6.3
Difference between average black and white typhoid death rates in cities with and without water filtration. Source: See text.

6.3 Estimating the Effects of Filtration on Black and White Disease Rates

To test the proposition that whites benefitted from water filtration disproportionately, variants on the following equations were estimated:

$$y_{it}^b = \mathbf{a}^b + \mathbf{t}^b + \beta^b FILTER_{it} + \varepsilon_{it}^b, \tag{6.1}$$

$$y_{it}^w = \mathbf{a}^w + \mathbf{t}^w + \beta^w FILTER_{it} + \varepsilon_{it}^w, \tag{6.2}$$

$$DIFF_{it} = \mathbf{a}^f + \mathbf{t}^f + \beta^f FILTER_{it} + \varepsilon_{it}^f, \tag{6.3}$$

where y_{it}^b is the black typhoid rate measured as deaths from typhoid per 100,000 persons in city i in year t and y_{it}^w is the rate for whites; $DIFF$ is either the ratio of, or the difference between, black and white typhoid rates in city i in year t; the **a**s are vectors of city dummies that control for fixed characteristics in each city i; the **t**s are vectors of time dummies that control for shocks common to all cities in period t; $FILTER$ is a filtration dummy that assumes a value of one if a water

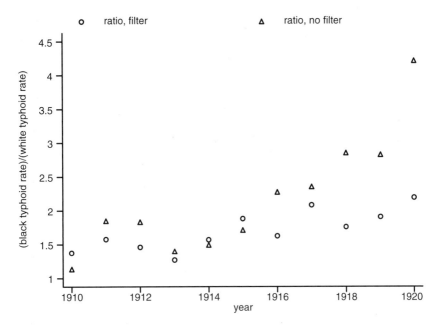

Figure 6.4
Ratio of average black and white typhoid death rates in cities with and without filters.
Source: See text.

filter was present in city i in year t, and zero otherwise; and the εs are random-error terms.

The variable of primary interest is *FILTER*. If blacks had limited access to local water systems, the introduction of filtration would have reduced white typhoid rates sharply but black rates only slightly, if at all. This hypothesis predicts the following coefficient estimates on *FILTER*: $\beta^b > \beta^w$ and $\beta^f > 0$. Before turning to the results, it is important to clarify the causal relationship between *FILTER* and black and white typhoid rates. Obviously cities with the highest typhoid rates had the strongest incentives to install water filters, and with cross-sectional data, this would necessitate the use of instrumental variables. However, with panel data, instrumental variables are neither necessary nor desirable, because *FILTER* and typhoid death rates were not simultaneously determined. Cities did not begin filtering when typhoid rates rose and stop filtering when they started to fall. The installation of a water filter was permanent. Moreover, installing a filter involved spending millions of dollars and typically required cities to overcome a series of bureaucratic, legal, and political hurdles. These included, but were not limited to, issuing new debt, lobbying state legislators for the authority to issue such debt, holding referendum votes to assess voter demand for expenditures and debt, and litigation with voters and city residents who opposed expenditures on filters. The legal institutions that determined how many hurdles the city had to overcome, as well as the height of those hurdles, were established by state constitutions decades earlier and varied across cities. This caused randomness in the timing of the installation of filters across cities.[2]

6.4   Results: Full Sample, North and South Subsamples

Table 6.3 contains the regression results for the full sample of cities. Although their coefficients are not given, all regressions include city and time dummies; regressions 2a–2d also include city-specific time trends. Regressions 1a–1d provide strong evidence against the hypothesis that cities systematically denied African Americans access to public water systems. The introduction of filtration reduced black typhoid rates by 22 deaths per 100,000 persons (a 53 percent reduction from the mean); it reduced white rates by a statistically insignificant 4.5 deaths per 100,000 persons (a 16 percent reduction from the mean); and it reduced the difference between white and black rates by about 18 deaths per 100,000 persons. If we compare the percentage reductions in typhoid rates by examining the ratio of black to white typhoid rates, the same conclusion emerges; filtration reduced the ratio by 47 percentage points (a 26 percent reduction from the mean). Except for those regarding the ratio,[3] the results are robust to the addition of city-specific time trends that control for unobserved city-level changes that might also have been driving down typhoid rates (see regressions 2a–2d).[4]

Table 6.4 shows the results for the South-alone subsample. In the South, the introduction of filtration reduced black typhoid rates by 22 deaths per 100,000 persons (a 46 percent reduction from the mean); it reduced white rates by a statistically insignificant 9 deaths per 100,000 persons (a 23 percent reduction from the mean); and it reduced the difference between white and black rates by about 12 deaths per 100,000 persons. If we compare the percentage reductions in typhoid rates by examining the ratio of black to white rates, the same conclusion emerges; filtration reduced the ratio by 33 percentage points (a 22 percent reduction from the mean) (see table 6.4, regressions 1a–1d). For the South, the results are sensitive to the addition of city-specific time

Table 6.3
Filtration and Typhoid in a Panel of Thirty-Three American Cities

Variable	Full sample, without trends				Full sample, with trends			
	1a	1b	1c	1d	2a	2b	2c	2d
	y^b	y^w	$y^b - y^w$	y^b/y^w	y^b	y^w	$y^b - y^w$	y^b/y^w
=1 if filter present	−22.4*	−4.50*	−17.9*	−0.468	−23.8*	−3.53	−20.2*	−0.339
	(5.13)	(1.59)	(4.45)	(2.20)	(5.76)	(3.70)	(5.46)	(0.279)
Year dummies	Yes	Yes	Yes	Yes	Yes	Yes	Yes	Yes
City dummies	Yes	Yes	Yes	Yes	Yes	Yes	Yes	Yes
City-specific trends	No	No	No	No	Yes	Yes	Yes	Yes
No. of observations	484	484	484	481	484	484	484	481
Adjusted R^2	0.549	0.610	0.291	0.207	0.587	0.650	0.314	0.281

Source: See text.
Notes: Standard errors are reported in parentheses. An asterisk indicates significant at the 10 percent level or higher, one-tailed test. Variables are as defined in table 6.2.

Table 6.4
Race, Typhoid, and Filtration in Southern Cities

Variable	South only, without trends				South only, with trends			
	1a	1b	1c	1d	2a	2b	2c	2d
	y^b	y^w	$y^b - y^w$	y^b/y^w	y^b	y^w	$y^b - y^w$	y^b/y^w
=1 if filter present	−21.5*	−9.24*	−12.3*	−0.332*	−6.57	5.77	−12.3	−0.116
	(6.17)	(5.32)	(6.14)	(0.267)	(9.23)	(7.82)	(9.61)	(0.406)
Year dummies	Yes	Yes	Yes	Yes	Yes	Yes	Yes	Yes
City dummies	Yes	Yes	Yes	Yes	Yes	Yes	Yes	Yes
City-specific time trends	No	No	No	No	Yes	Yes	Yes	Yes
No. of observations	236	236	236	234	236	236	236	234
Adjusted R^2	0.514	0.517	0.062	0.207	0.549	0.567	0.252	0.106

Source: See text.
Notes: Standard errors are reported in parentheses. An asterisk indicates significant at the 10 percent level or higher, one-tailed test. Variables are as defined in table 6.2. The cities coded as southern are Birmingham, Ala.; Charleston, S.C.; New Orleans, La.; San Antonio, Texas; Atlanta, Ga.; Jacksonville, Fla.; Memphis, Tenn.; Nashville, Tenn.; Norfolk, Va.; Richmond, Va.; Augusta, Ga.; Charlotte, N.C.; Lynchburg, Va.; Montgomery, Ala.; and Savannah, Ga.

trends.[5] The addition of these trends changes the sign on the filtration coefficient for whites and increases the standard errors on the estimates for blacks. Although the coefficient estimates are insignificant, they still suggest that blacks benefitted more than whites from the installation of filters (see table 6.4, regressions 2a–2d). Table 6.5 reports the results for cities outside the South. These results are identical to those for the full sample and require no elaboration.

6.5   Exploring the Effects of Residential Segregation

If the findings for Memphis and Savannah generalize, evidence of unequal access to public water systems should become stronger if the sample is restricted to highly segregated cities. To test this proposition, the analysis that follows employed a well-known index of segregation, the index of isolation.[6] As noted in chapter 4, this index varies from 0 to 1, with 1 indicating complete segregation. The cities in the panel are arrayed according to the value of their isolation index as of 1910. There are six cities (Montgomery, Alabama; Augusta, Georgia; Savannah, Georgia; Newport, Kentucky; Charlotte, North Carolina; and Lynchburg, Virginia) for which the index is not available, and these cities are dropped from the analysis. The remaining cities are divided into two subsamples as follows: Cities with an index greater than or equal to the median value of the isolation index (0.085) fall into one subsample and are called segregated cities, while cities with an index value less than the median fall into the other subsample and are called integrated cities. The regression models specified in Eqs. (6.1)–(6.3) are then applied to the integrated and segregated subsamples.

Table 6.6 contains the results for integrated cities. Once again there is evidence that blacks benefitted from water filtration and that they benefitted more than whites. The introduction of filtration reduced black typhoid death rates by 25 deaths per 100,000 persons (a 57 percent reduction from the mean); it reduced white rates by 5 deaths per 100,000 persons (a 19 percent reduction from the mean); and it reduced the difference between white and black rates by about 19 deaths per 100,000 persons. If we compare the percentage reductions in typhoid rates by examining the ratio of black to white rates, the same conclusion emerges; filtration reduced the ratio by 53 percentage points (a 26 percent reduction from the mean). The results are robust to the addition of city-specific time trends (see table 6.6, regressions 2a–2d).

Table 6.5
Race, Typhoid, and Filtration in Cities Outside the South

	non-South only, without trends				non-South only, with trends			
	1a	1b	1c	1d	2a	2b	2c	2d
Variable	y^b	y^w	$y^b - y^w$	y^b / y^w	y^b	y^w	$y^b - y^w$	y^b / y^w
=1 if filter present	−18.9*	−5.92*	−13.1*	−0.798*	−27.2*	−7.84*	−19.4*	−0.417
	(6.16)	(1.97)	(5.61)	(0.380)	(6.40)	(1.92)	(6.22)	(0.419)
Year dummies	Yes	Yes	Yes	Yes	Yes	Yes	Yes	Yes
City dummies	Yes	Yes	Yes	Yes	Yes	Yes	Yes	Yes
City-specific time trends	No	No	No	No	Yes	Yes	Yes	Yes
No. of observations	248	248	248	247	248	248	248	247
Adjusted R^2	0.653	0.817	0.447	0.170	0.724	0.871	0.447	0.253

Source: See text.

Notes: Standard errors are reported in parentheses. An asterisk indicates significant at the 10 percent level or higher, one-tailed test. Variables are as defined in table 6.2. The cities coded as non-South are Cincinnati, Ohio; Columbus, Ohio; Los Angeles, Calif.; New York, N.Y.; Pittsburgh, Pa.; San Francisco, Calif.; Washington, D.C.; Wilmington, Del.; Baltimore, Md.; Boston, Mass.; Chicago, Ill.; Covington, Ky.; Kansas City, Mo.; Louisville, Ky.; Philadelphia, Pa.; St. Louis, Mo.; and Newport, R.I.

Table 6.6
Race, Typhoid, and Filtration in Integrated Cities

Variable	Integrated cities, without trends				Integrated cities, with trends			
	1a y^b	1b y^w	1c $y^b - y^w$	1d y^b / y^w	2a y^b	2b y^w	2c $y^b - y^w$	2d y^b / y^w
=1 if filter present	−24.5*	−5.10*	−19.4*	−0.530*	−26.1*	−6.66*	−19.4*	−0.233
	(6.97)	(3.08)	(6.04)	(0.408)	(8.91)	(3.97)	(8.02)	(0.542)
Year dummies	Yes	Yes	Yes	Yes	Yes	Yes	Yes	Yes
City dummies	Yes	Yes	Yes	Yes	Yes	Yes	Yes	Yes
City-specific time trends	No	No	No	No	Yes	Yes	Yes	Yes
No. of observations	190	190	190	190	190	190	190	190
Adjusted R^2	0.635	0.756	0.284	0.216	0.701	0.797	0.455	0.308

Source: See text.
Notes: Standard errors are reported in parentheses. An asterisk indicates significant at the 10 percent level or higher, one-tailed test. Variables are as defined in table 6.2. The cities coded as integrated are Birmingham, Ala.; Charleston, S.C.; Cincinnati, Ohio; Columbus, Ohio; Los Angeles, Calif.; New Orleans, La.; New York, N.Y.; Pittsburgh, Pa.; San Antonio, Texas; San Francisco, Calif.; Washington, D.C.; and Wilmington, Del.

Table 6.7 reports the results for segregated cities. Here there is only modest evidence of absolute improvement in typhoid rates, for either blacks or whites, and only weak evidence that blacks benefitted disproportionately. The introduction of filtration reduced black typhoid death rates by 7 deaths per 100,000 persons (a 20 percent reduction from the mean); it reduced white rates by less than 1 death per 100,000 persons; and it reduced the difference between white and black rates by 7 deaths per 100,000 persons. If we compare the percentage reductions in typhoid rates by examining the ratio of black to white rates, we find the ratio might have risen by 3 percentage points following the introduction of filtration.[7] The addition of city-specific time trends strengthens the evidence in favor of filtration reducing absolute and relative levels of typhoid for blacks, but not by very much (see table 6.7, regressions 2a–2d).

A comparison of the results for integrated (table 6.6) and segregated cities (table 6.7) suggests that the findings for Memphis and Savannah generalize. There was much more absolute and relative improvement in typhoid death rates for blacks in cities with relatively low levels of residential segregation than in those with high levels. For example, in segregated cities, point estimates suggest that the ratio of black to white typhoid death rates did not fall after filtration, while in integrated cities it fell by 53 percentage points. There is, however, one puzzling finding. Reductions in typhoid death rates for whites are also much smaller in segregated cities than in integrated cities. It is not immediately obvious why this would have been so. This puzzling finding is resolved by the regression results reported in the next section.

6.6   Measuring the Size of Disease Spillovers

The panel data can also be used to measure the size of disease spillovers between black and white households. The simplest procedure would be to regress the white typhoid rate in city i in year t against the black typhoid rate in the same year. Not surprisingly, if one performs this exercise, there is strong evidence that white and black typhoid death rates moved together over time. Specifically, after including city and time dummies, the coefficient on contemporaneous black typhoid rates is 0.281 with a t-statistic of 10.2. This, however, only establishes that a strong correlation existed between contemporaneous black and white typhoid death rates. It does not tell us whether the correlation existed because there were spillovers or because the same external and

Table 6.7
Race, Typhoid, and Filtration in Segregated Cities

Variable	Segregated cities, without trends				Segregated cities, with trends			
	1a	1b	1c	1d	2a	2b	2c	2d
	y^b	y^w	$y^b - y^w$	y^b / y^w	y^b	y^w	$y^b - y^w$	y^b / y^w
=1 if filter present	−7.30*	−0.029	−7.27*	0.033	−8.40*	−5.41*	−2.99*	−0.007
	(4.63)	(3.49)	(4.14)	(0.256)	(5.46)	(4.32)	(5.43)	(0.342)
Year dummies	Yes	Yes	Yes	Yes	Yes	Yes	Yes	Yes
City dummies	Yes	Yes	Yes	Yes	Yes	Yes	Yes	Yes
City-specific time trends	No	No	No	No	Yes	Yes	Yes	Yes
No. of observations	206	206	206	206	206	206	206	206
Adjusted R^2	0.580	0.647	0.249	0.138	0.681	0.706	0.295	0.163

Source: See text.
Notes: Standard errors are reported in parentheses. An asterisk indicates significant at the 10 percent level or higher, one-tailed test. Variables are as defined in table 6.2. The cities coded as segregated are Atlanta, Ga.; Baltimore, Md.; Boston, Mass.; Chicago, Ill.; Covington, Ky.; Jacksonville, Fla.; Kansas City, Mo.; Louisville, Ky.; Memphis, Tenn.; Nashville, Tenn.; Norfolk, Va.; Philadelphia, Pa.; Richmond, Va.; and St. Louis, Mo.

unidentified (city-specific) shocks that affected black typhoid rates also affected white rates. A related concern is the potential simultaneity between white and black rates. A crude way of controlling for unidentified shocks is to add a lag of the white typhoid rate; and a crude way of controlling for the potential simultaneity between black and white typhoid rates is to replace the contemporaneous black rate with the lagged black rate.

Table 6.8 shows the results of seven models in which current white typhoid rates were regressed against lagged black and lagged white typhoid rates. In the first four regressions, if after controlling for lagged white rates one finds a significant positive relationship between lagged black rates and current white rates, this would suggest that outbreaks of typhoid among African-American households sometimes spread to white households. Regressing the current white typhoid rate against the lagged black rate, there appears to be a strong correlation between black and white typhoid rates. However, after adding a lag of the white typhoid rate, the coefficient on the lagged black rate shrinks and becomes statistically insignificant (compare regressions 1 and 2). A possible objection to this procedure is that spillovers might have arisen only during unusually severe outbreaks of typhoid fever. To address this possibility, a dummy variable indicating especially large shocks was added to the regressions. The shock dummy assumes a value of one whenever typhoid rates exceed 150 deaths per 100,000 persons (the top 2.5 percent of the distribution), and zero otherwise. Using this procedure, stronger evidence of spillovers emerges; (lagged) black typhoid shocks have a significant effect on current white rates, even after controlling for (lagged) white typhoid shocks (see regression 3).

Given typhoid's long incubation period and the fact that it peaked during the months of September, October, and November, one might also want to consider a more involved lag structure. Regression 4 addresses this concern by including typhoid death rates lagged 1 and 2 years. Using this procedure, additional evidence of spillovers emerges; lagged black rates have a significant effect on current whites rates, even after controlling for lagged white rates. A comparison of the results in table 6.8 with those in table 6.3 reveals the following: After controlling for spillovers from black to white households, the coefficient on filtration is one-quarter the size it would be without such controls and is (highly) statistically insignificant. This is a startling finding. It suggests that most of the benefits whites derived from the introduction of water filtration were indirect and originated from the reduced

Table 6.8
Spillovers in the Panel Data

Regression	y_{-1}^b	y_{-2}^b	=1: $y_{-1}^b > 150$	y_{-1}^w	y_{-2}^w	=1: $y_{-1}^w > 150$	=1 if filter	Adj. R^2
Full sample								
1 y_0^w	0.149* (4.76)	...	...	...	...	...	-1.01 (0.341)	0.63
2 y_0^w	0.035 (1.10)	...	...	0.390* (7.76)	...	...	-1.75 (0.630)	0.68
3 y_0^w	0.015 (0.395)	...	13.2* (2.09)	0.229* (4.09)	...	57.2* (5.04)	-0.723 (0.270)	0.71
4 y_0^w	0.062 (1.76)	0.076* (2.38)	...	0.348* (6.55)	-0.019 (0.363)	...	-1.01 (0.355)	0.69
5 y_0^b	0.230* (4.30)	-0.001 (0.020)	...	0.278* (3.44)	0.180* (2.23)	...	-10.8* (2.50)	0.65
Integrated cities only								
6 y_0^w	0.080* (2.14)	...	...	0.273* (3.26)	...	...	-1.48 (0.51)	0.82
7 y_0^w	...	...	17.6* (2.98)	...	...	-25.5* (3.48)	-2.79 (0.92)	0.77
Segregated cities only								
8 y_0^w	0.053 (0.80)	...	...	0.201* (2.30)	...	...	1.23 (0.35)	0.65
9 y_0^w	...	...	3.79 (0.56)	...	...	Dropped	0.24 (0.01)	0.67

Source: See text.

Notes: All regressions include city and time period dummies. An asterisk indicates significant at the 10 percent level or higher, one-tailed test. y^b and y^w are as defined in table 6.2. In regression 9, the dummy variable (=1: $y_{-1}^w > 150$) is dropped from the estimation because there is no variation. In segregated cities, white typhoid rates never rose above 150 deaths per 100,000 persons, and so the dummy variable (=1: $y_{-1}^w > 150$) assumes a value of zero throughout. t-Statistics are in parentheses.

risk of typhoid fever spreading from black to white households. The direct benefits of filtration to whites were small. In contrast, blacks realized substantial direct benefits in terms of reduced typhoid death rates, even after controlling for the spillovers that ran from white to black households (see regression 5).

Disease Spillovers and Segregation

The finding that whites gained from water filtration primarily through a reduced risk of typhoid fever spreading from black to white households can help resolve the puzzling result that whites in segregated cities benefitted very little from the installation of filters. (Recall that in segregated cities there was evidence that whites gained very little from filtration, while in integrated cities they benefitted substantially.) It is likely that disease spillovers, at least between blacks and whites, were larger in integrated than in segregated cities. Assuming that this is true, and remembering that whites gained from water filtration only to the extent that it reduced disease spillovers from blacks to whites, whites would have gained little from filtration in segregated cities because in these cities there were few disease spillovers to begin with. In other words, filtration could not have reduced white typhoid death rates in segregated cities because disease spillovers were already low in those cities, and that was the primary avenue through which filtration reduced white typhoid rates. Put yet another way, whites in segregated cities did not benefit from filtration because segregation was already protecting them against disease spillovers from blacks.

The regression results in table 6.8 corroborate this line of thought. The bottom two sections of the table report the results of regressions run separately for integrated and segregated cities. Consider first the results for integrated cities, which are reported in regressions 6 and 7. Notice that there is evidence of disease spillovers; lagged black typhoid rates increase white typhoid rates, even after controlling for lagged white typhoid rates. Furthermore, the estimated coefficients on the filtration dummy are made insignificant once controls for disease spillovers are added. Indeed, the coefficients on filtration in regressions 6 and 7 are one-quarter to one-half the size of the coefficient reported in regressions 1b and 2b in table 6.6. As with the full sample, whites in integrated cities realized benefits from filtration only to the extent that it reduced disease spillovers from blacks to whites. The results, however, are very different for segregated cities. As regressions 8 and 9 show, there is no evidence of disease spillovers in segregated cities. Note that in regression 9 unusually large typhoid rates for whites have been dropped from the estimate. This is because there is no change in this variable; in segregated cities white typhoid rates never rose above 150 deaths per 100,000 persons.

6.7 Conclusions

The econometric results presented here are quite strong. In most cities, the installation of water filters benefitted both blacks and whites in terms of disease reduction, and in the full sample of cities, as well as in several subsamples, blacks actually benefitted more than whites. As shown further in chapter 7, these are statistically robust findings that contradict the idea that blacks were systematically denied access to public water and sewer systems. There is, however, evidence that blacks gained much less from filtration in segregated than in integrated cities, suggesting that segregation facilitated efforts to deny blacks service. Beyond this, there were large disease spillovers from the black to white communities, and these spillovers were so large that most of the benefits that whites realized from water filtration were indirect. Filtration reduced the incidence of typhoid in black communities and this in turn reduced the number of black-to-white disease transmissions. Disease spillovers were much lower in segregated than in integrated cities, and as a result whites garnered few indirect benefits from filtration in segregated cities and filtration had little, if any, direct effect on white disease rates in these cities.

As I noted in my discussion of the econometric results, however, there is a caveat to all of this. Some of my findings are sensitive to how I control for prefiltration time trends, and to what metric I use to measure disparities in disease rates: the difference between, or the ratio of, black and white typhoid death rates. Both of these issues are fully addressed in chapter 7.

7   Verification

7.1   Introduction

The econometric results in chapter 6 are critical for my larger arguments about disease spillovers, segregation, and racial parity in access to public water and sewer facilities. Hence these results deserve close scrutiny, both empirically and conceptually. This chapter provides such scrutiny. In particular, it explores the robustness of my empirical findings to alternative estimation strategies. It expressly states the assumptions that underlie the statistical work in chapter 6 and tests the validity of these assumptions. Finally, it explores the reliability of the data used in chapter 6.

7.2   How to Estimate the Benefits of Water Filtration

In this section I discuss various econometric techniques for estimating the benefits of water filtration. I begin with a discussion of a hypothetical example. The purpose of this stylized case is to reveal clearly and precisely the assumptions that underlie the empirical work in chapter 6. To give this hypothetical discussion some empirical substance, the chapter provides a detailed case study of typhoid fever rates in Washington, D.C. This study is not meant to establish any substantive historical argument, but instead is meant to identify and suggest competing econometric approaches. After describing these various approaches, I apply them to the data used in chapter 6 to see if the results withstand reasonable respecifications of the econometric model.

A Stylized Example

To measure the effects of water filtration on health, a common practice is to compare typhoid rates before and after the introduction of water

treatment. Such comparisons invariably show that typhoid rates are
significantly lower after treatment than before.[1] One problem with this
approach, however, is that typhoid rates might have fallen even without the installation of water filters. This is particularly true of American cities during the late nineteenth and early twentieth centuries,
when the germ theory of disease grew more popular and people
changed their behavior accordingly.[2] In concrete terms, as people
learned what caused typhoid, they probably began to take more personal precautions. Failure to control for this effect might lead one to
overestimate the benefits of public investments in filtration or chlorination. In chapter 6 I controlled for such preexisting trends by adding
city-specific time trends to the regression models, a standard practice when using panel data. Unfortunately, this otherwise standard
technique might generate its own, and perhaps more serious, set of
problems.

To illustrate, consider figure 7.1, which plots typhoid rates in some
hypothetical city from time t_0 onward. This city installs a water filter
at time t^*. Note that prior to the installation of a water filter at t^*, typhoid rates follow a wavelike pattern around a secular downward
trend labeled "true pre-existing trend." The assumption that typhoid
rates exhibit this wavelike pattern is both important and historically
accurate. The natural progression of typhoid was such that after a large
outbreak, the weak and frail were quickly killed off and those remain-

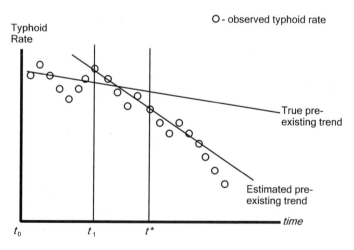

Figure 7.1
Estimating secular trends in typhoid death rates in a hypothetical city. Source: See text.

ing either had innate immunities to the disease or were particularly vigilant about their sanitary practices. As a result, typhoid rates would fall sharply and would remain low until a new population of vulnerable persons arrived, or until some in the remaining population became lax in their sanitary practices. Typhoid rates would then spike again, and the same patterns would be repeated.[3] As will be made clear in a later section of this chapter, one can observe such wavelike patterns in most cities prior to the installation of water filters.

Suppose now that we want to identify the effects of water filtration on disease rates, net of any secular downward trends that were independent of filtration. Econometrically, the goal would be to separate the effects of the true preexisting downward trend in figure 7.1 from the effects of water filtration. If we simply compared the average typhoid rate before and after filtration, we would overestimate the benefits of filtration because its effects would be conflated with those of the secular downward trend. A reasonable and obvious solution here would appear to be to run a regression that includes an overall time trend as well as a dummy variable for filtration. (As noted earlier, if we had a panel of cities, as in chapter 6, this would amount to including city-specific time trends along with time period and city dummies.)

Unfortunately, in a world where historical data are scarce and become more scarce the further back in time we go, this is one case where the cure might be worse than the disease. To see this, suppose that the data for this hypothetical city did not extend back in time past t_1, so that all observations between t_0 and t_1 are unavailable. If we ran a regression that included a time trend and filtration dummy only on data after t_1, the estimated trend line would look like the line labeled "estimated pre-existing trend" in figure 7.1. The resulting coefficient estimate on the filtration dummy would be biased against finding any evidence that filtration reduced disease rates. The reason that the estimated trend is so different from the actual trend is that we are picking up the effects of the short-term oscillations in typhoid rates and confusing these effects with the actual trend. While this is a contrived scenario, a case study of Washington suggests that this is no small matter, and that the way one controls for preexisting trends matters.

Typhoid Fever and Water Filtration in Washington

Figure 7.2 plots the death rate from typhoid fever in Washington from 1895 to 1925. The city installed a slow-sand filter in 1906, a coagulation

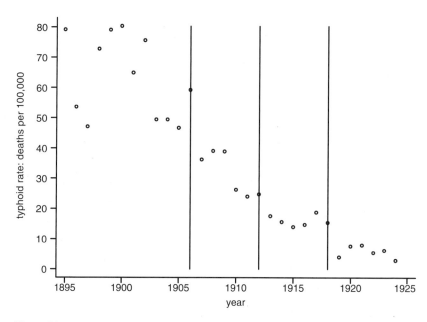

Figure 7.2
Typhoid death rates in Washington, D.C., 1895–1925. The vertical lines indicate improvements in the city's water purification systems. Sources: Fuller, "Water-Works," p. 1220; U.S. Bureau of Census, *Mortality Statistics*, various years; U.S. Bureau of Census, *General Statistics of Cities*. Data prepared by Center for Population Economics, University of Chicago.

filter in 1911, and began chlorinating its water supply around 1918. The installation of the filters and the onset of chlorination are indicated by vertical lines. Two important patterns are evident in figure 7.2. First, before the installation of Washington's first water filter, typhoid death rates in the city exhibit a wavelike pattern. The data trend sharply downward between 1895 and 1898, spike upward between 1898 and 1901, stabilize briefly, and then trend sharply downward again between 1904 and 1906. Second, the raw data suggest that filtration and chlorination substantially reduced typhoid rates in Washington. Drops in typhoid death rates and changes in trends seem to be highly correlated with the installation of filters and the introduction of chlorination.

To identify the benefits of water purification more precisely, one might compare typhoid rates before and after the installation of the filters, and, as explained earlier, this is exactly what most previous studies do. A simple way to implement such an experiment is to regress typhoid rates against a series of dummy variables that indicate the presence of filtration or chlorination. The results of this regression are shown in table 7.1 (see regression 1). The coefficient estimates suggest that the installation of the first water filter in 1906 reduced typhoid death rates by 26 points, a 41 percent reduction from the mean rate in the pre-1906 period. The combined effects of both filters and chlorination was to reduce typhoid death rates in the city by 58 points, a 91 percent reduction from their pre-1906 mean. In effect, this regression is a means test and implements the same procedure as Edward Meeker's widely cited study of the health benefits of water and sewer systems. In terms of the empirical work in chapter 6, this regression would be (almost) equivalent to the results without city-specific trends.[4]

If, however, an overall time trend is added to the regression, the results change dramatically. In absolute value, the estimated coefficients are about one-third the size of the coefficients in the first regression, and are significant at only low levels (see regression 2). If one adopts a more elaborate estimation procedure that allows changes in both slope and intercept terms, the results do not appear to strengthen the case for filtration (see regression 3). Restricting the coefficient on the trend term to be −1.64, the estimate for the pre-1906 period, the case for filtration is made stronger, although the estimates on the filtration and chlorination dummies are still half the size of the estimates in the first regression (compare regressions 1 and 4).

A reasonable objection to regressions 2–4 is that each of them uses a linear function to approximate, and control for, an essentially nonlinear relationship. To address this objection, I transform the year variable by its cosine and include the cosine as a regressor. Adding the cosine to the regression allows typhoid rates to follow a wavelike pattern. This transformation fits the data well and is significant in regressions 5 and 6. Moreover, including the cosine in the regression reduces the estimated absolute value of the coefficient on year by 38 percent, from 1.84 to 1.14 (compare regressions 2 and 6). In other words, controlling for short-term oscillations in typhoid rates significantly reduces the magnitude of the secular downward trend in rates. The impact of this control on the estimated effect of filtration is substantial. In absolute terms, the estimated benefits of filtration are increased by as much as 84 percent (compare again regressions 2 and 6).

The most-preferred estimates of the benefits of filtration are those derived from regression 8. In this regression the coefficient on year is restricted to be −1.045 and the coefficient on the cosine of year is restricted to be −11.25. These restrictions are based on the results from

Table 7.1
Water Filtration and Typhoid Rates in Washington, D.C.

	1	2	3	4	5	6	7	8
				Dependent variable (pre-1906 mean = 63.5)				
Typhoid: deaths per 100,000								
=1 if 1906 filter present[a]	−26.2*	−10.6	8,116.4*	−12.3*	−27.0*	−17.1*	...	−18.5*
	(5.40)	(8.00)	(4,698)	(4.85)	(4.84)	(8.49)		(5.12)
=1 if 1911 filter present[b]	−46.2*	−18.7	−1,354.1	−21.6*	−47.1*	−29.8*	...	−31.9*
	(5.15)	(12.1)	(3,873)	(4.62)	(4.61)	(13.1)		(4.88)
=1 if 1918 chlorination[c]	−57.8*	−18.4	−2,505.6	−22.5*	−58.4*	−33.8*	...	−36.3*
	(5.41)	(16.7)	(4,735)	(4.85)	(4.84)	(18.2)		(5.12)
Year	...	−1.83*	−1.64*	−1.64[d]	...	−1.14	−1.05	−1.05[d]
		(0.740)	(0.913)			(0.810)	(1.17)	
Year × 1906 filter	...	...	−4.29*	...	...	...	...	...
			(2.46)					
Year × 1911 filter	...	...	0.70	...	...	...	...	...
			(2.03)					
Year × 1918 chlorine	...	...	1.29	...	...	...	...	...
			(2.46)					
Cosine (year)	...	...	...	...	−6.83*	−4.95*	−11.3*	−11.3[d]
					(2.88)	(2.79)	(5.37)	
Adjusted R^2	0.829	0.857	0.862	...	0.863	0.868	0.309	...
No. of observations	30	30	30	30	30	30	11	30

Source: See text.
Notes: Standard errors are in parentheses. An asterisk indicates significant at the 5 percent level or higher (one-tailed test).
[a] Assumes a value of one if year greater than 1906 and less than 1912.
[b] Assumes a value of one if year greater than 1911 and less than 1919.
[c] Assumes a value of one if year greater than 1918.
[d] Fixed by assumption.

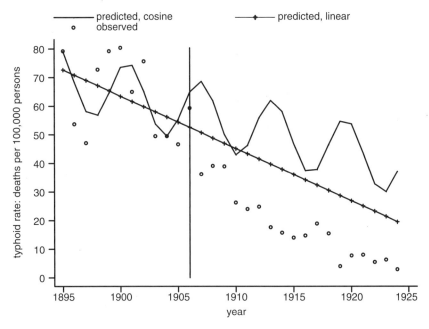

Figure 7.3
Alternative trend estimators in Washington, D.C. The straight line with plus signs represents the estimated prefiltration trend using a simple linear estimator. The line without symbols and following a wavelike pattern is the estimated prefiltration trend using a combined linear and cosine estimator. Source: See text.

regression 7, which is estimated for data during the prefiltration period. That is, regression 7 is estimated with the 11 years of data before 1906. Unlike earlier specifications, this regression identifies the secular trend in typhoid death rates that was independent of both filtration and short-term oscillations in typhoid death rates. After the coefficients on the year and cosine terms are restricted to their prefiltration values, the estimated benefit of filtration is large. In particular, the estimates suggest that the installation of the first filter in 1906 reduced typhoid rates by 29 percent from their mean, prefiltration level. The estimated collective effect of filtration and chlorination is that these measures reduced typhoid rates by 57 percent (see regression 8).

It is useful to illustrate the differences in these estimation techniques graphically. To this end, figure 7.3 plots the actual and predicted typhoid rates if no filters or chlorination systems had been installed. There are two predicted series. The first series, which is a straight line with plus signs, plots predicted typhoid death rates using a linear estimation technique, akin to what is reported in regression 2. The second series, which resembles a series of sine waves with an overall downward trend, plots predicted rates using a cosine estimator that also allows a linear trend, akin to what is reported in regression 8. It is clear from the graph that the second estimation technique does a much better job of approximating the true relationship between time and typhoid death rates during the prefiltration period than the first linear estimation procedure. Notice also that in contrast to the crude linear estimation, the cosine estimation predicts that in the absence of filtration, typhoid rates would have continued to exhibit a wavelike pattern. Notice too that the (prefiltration) secular trend implied by the cosine estimation is not as steep as the trend implied by the crude linear estimation.

Prefiltration Waves in Other Cities

The wavelike pattern observed in Washington is not unique to that city. Similar patterns can be observed in figures 2.2 and 2.3, which plot typhoid rates in Philadelphia and Chicago. Regressing typhoid death rates against time during the *prefiltration* period in both of these cities confirms the visual inspection. A simple linear trend line does a poor job of approximating the relationship between typhoid and time during the years before filtration, although its accuracy improves the more data one has. As table 7.2 shows, the linear time trend alone does a very poor job of predicting changes in typhoid death rates in Chicago. The cosine, on the other hand, is significant and reduces the estimated coefficient on the time trend by 20 percent (see regressions 1 and 2). In contrast, in Philadelphia, the time trend alone performs much better, and adding the cosine of the time period does not significantly alter the estimated linear trend. Notice that the tangent of the time period does much better than the cosine in controlling for Philadelphia's unusual wavelike pattern, although including the tangent does not alter the estimated slope of the trend line (compare regressions 3 and 5).

The sharp contrast between the results for Chicago and Philadelphia is worth exploring. One likely explanation is that the number of observations for prefiltration Philadelphia is nearly double the number for prefiltration Chicago. As a result, it is easier to sort out long-term trends from short-term oscillations in Philadelphia than in Chicago. This explanation suggests that with a sufficient number of observations, the need to control for waves and spikes in typhoid rates is

Table 7.2
Trend Estimators in Chicago and Philadelphia

	Chicago		Philadelphia		
	1	2	3	4	5
Typhoid: deaths per 100,000	Dependent variable		Dependent variable		
Year	1.47	1.18	−0.704*	−0.703*	−0.702*
	(2.29)	(2.09)	(0.334)	(0.340)	(0.321)
Cosine (year)	. . .	25.0*	. . .	−0.436	. . .
		(13.0)		(3.90)	
Tangent (year)	. . .	. . .	. . .	. . .	0.957*
					(0.546)
Adjusted R^2	−0.044	0.136	0.113	0.078	0.179
No. of observations	15	15	28	28	28

Source: See text.
Notes: Standard errors are in parentheses. An asterisk indicates significant at the 5 percent level or higher (one-tailed test).

greatly diminished. Also, this explanation is worth remembering because in a later analysis it is used to justify the choice of some econometric specifications over others.

Implications for Econometric Analysis

At this point it is convenient to specify how all of this bears on the empirical work in chapter 6. Recall that in chapter 6 I assembled data on typhoid death rates for a panel of thirty-three cities from across the United States. For most cities the rates were observed for 15 years, from 1906 through 1920. I also collected data on the installation of water purification systems in each of these cities over the same period. With these data, the typhoid death rates were regressed against a dummy variable that indicated the presence of a water purification system. This procedure estimates the average effect of water filtration and chlorination on typhoid rates. Following convention, I included year dummies to control for time-related shocks common to all cities, and city dummies to control for fixed effects specific to each city. I also included city-specific trends in typhoid death rates to control for any secular trends in disease rates that were independent of water purification. However, the experience of Washington suggests that including city-specific time trends might generate results that significantly understate the benefits of water purification.

I have adopted three different estimation strategies to address the concern about secular trends and the possibility that short-term oscillations around those trends might bias estimates of the benefits of filtration. The first strategy is to include a single trend term that is common to all cities, rather than including a separate trend term for each city. The rationale for using this strategy is based on the contrasting findings for Chicago and Philadelphia in the previous section. Recall that these findings suggested that as the number of observations increases, the importance of controlling for short-term oscillations falls. This observation seems particularly relevant in the context of panel data analysis where typhoid rates in a particular year will be an average of many cities. Because it averages across the experience of multiple cities, the use of a single, overall time trend will not be unduly influenced by sharp oscillations in disease rates in a particular city.

The second empirical strategy is to directly control for the wavelike patterns specific to each city. That is, the regressions include both a linear city-specific time trend and a transformed city-specific trend that controls for wavelike movements. The third strategy is to run the regressions with and without city-specific time trends and then argue that the results with trends should be interpreted as lower-bound estimates of the benefits of filtration and those without as upper-bound estimates.

In chapter 6, I followed the third empirical strategy and reported results with and without city-specific time trends. In this chapter I replicate the regressions from chapter 6, except that this time I use the first (single overall time trend) and second (direct controls for city-specific waves) empirical strategies. The results are given in tables 7.3 through 7.7. All of the results are robust to these alternative estimation strategies, and if anything, the results in this chapter are stronger, in terms of supporting my larger thesis, than those reported in chapter 6.

7.3   Measuring Interracial Disparities: Ratios or Differences?

There are numerous studies in economics, demography, sociology, and history that use racial disparities in outcomes to isolate discrimination, or at least unequal treatment. Following these studies, chapter 6 used disparities in disease rates to isolate evidence of unequal access to public water and sewer lines. The intuition behind using disease rates is straightforward. If only white households had access to public water and sewer lines, the installation of public water filters would have

Table 7.3
Filtration and Typhoid in a Panel of Thirty-Three American Cities: Further Tests

Variable	Full sample, with single time trend				Full sample, with city-specific "waves"			
	1a	1b	1c	1d	2a	2b	2c	2d
	y^b	y^w	$y^b - y^w$	y^b/y^w	y^b	y^w	$y^b - y^w$	y^b/y^w
=1 if filter present	−22.4*	−4.50*	−17.9*	−0.468*	−22.7*	−4.14	−18.6*	−0.428*
	(4.37)	(2.83)	(4.03)	(0.213)	(6.02)	(3.89)	(5.61)	(0.294)
Overall time trend	−1.46*	−1.28*	−0.180*	−0.050	No	No	No	No
	(0.824)	(0.535)	(0.760)	(0.824)				
Year dummies	Yes	Yes	Yes	Yes	Yes	Yes	Yes	Yes
City dummies	Yes	Yes	Yes	Yes	Yes	Yes	Yes	Yes
City-specific time trends	No	No	No	No	Yes	Yes	Yes	Yes
City-specific "waves"	No	No	No	No	Yes	Yes	Yes	Yes
No. of observations	484	484	484	481	484	484	484	481
Adjusted R^2	0.549	0.610	0.291	0.207	0.591	0.647	0.342	0.280

Source: See text.
Notes: Standard errors are reported in parentheses. An asterisk indicates significant at the 10 percent level or higher, one-tailed test. Variables are as defined in table 6.2.

Table 7.4
Race, Typhoid, and Filtration in Southern Cities: Further Tests

Variable	South only, with single time trend				South only, with city-specific "waves"			
	1a	1b	1c	1d	2a	2b	2c	2d
	y^b	y^w	$y^b - y^w$	y^b/y^w	y^b	y^w	$y^b - y^w$	y^b/y^w
=1 if filter present	−21.5*	−9.24*	−12.3*	−0.332	−7.88	4.24	−12.1	−0.174
	(6.17)	(5.32)	(6.14)	(0.267)	(9.89)	(8.11)	(10.1)	(0.430)
Overall time trend	−3.67*	−1.24*	−2.43*	−0.012	No	No	No	No
	(0.626)	(0.540)	(0.624)	(0.626)				
Year dummies	Yes	Yes	Yes	Yes	Yes	Yes	Yes	Yes
City dummies	Yes	Yes	Yes	Yes	Yes	Yes	Yes	Yes
City-specific time trends	No	No	No	No	Yes	Yes	Yes	Yes
City-specific "waves"	No	No	No	No	Yes	Yes	Yes	Yes
No. of observations	236	236	236	234	236	236	236	234
Adjusted R^2	0.514	0.517	0.264	0.062	0.530	0.577	0.246	0.104

Source: See text.
Notes: Standard errors are reported in parentheses. An asterisk indicates significant at the 10 percent level or higher, one-tailed test. Variables are as defined in table 6.2.

Table 7.5
Race, Typhoid, and Filtration in Cities Outside the South: Further Tests

	non-South, with single time trend				non-South, with city-specific "waves"			
	1a	1b	1c	1d	2a	2b	2c	2d
Variable	y^b	y^w	$y^b - y^w$	y^b/y^w	y^b	y^w	$y^b - y^w$	y^b/y^w
=1 if filter present	−19.0*	−5.93*	−13.1*	−0.798*	−22.1*	−7.56*	−14.5*	−0.386
	(6.16)	(1.97)	(5.61)	(0.380)	(6.14)	(1.93)	(6.01)	(0.446)
Overall time trend	−1.92*	−1.14*	−0.781	0.074	No	No	No	No
	(0.807)	(0.258)	(0.734)	(0.050)				
Year dummies	Yes	Yes	Yes	Yes	Yes	Yes	Yes	Yes
City dummies	Yes	Yes	Yes	Yes	Yes	Yes	Yes	Yes
City-specific time trends	No	No	No	No	Yes	Yes	Yes	Yes
City-specific "waves"	No	No	No	No	Yes	Yes	Yes	Yes
No. of observations	248	248	248	247	248	248	248	247
Adjusted R^2	0.653	0.817	0.391	0.170	0.772	0.884	0.342	0.245

Source: See text.
Notes: Standard errors are reported in parentheses. An asterisk indicates significant at the 10 percent level or higher, one-tailed test. Variables are as defined in table 6.2.

Table 7.6
Race, Typhoid, and Filtration in Integrated Cities: Further Tests

Variable	Integrated cities, with single time trend				Integrated cities, with city-specific "waves"			
	1a	1b	1c	1d	2a	2b	2c	2d
	y^b	y^w	$y^b - y^w$	y^b/y^w	y^b	y^w	$y^b - y^w$	y^b/y^w
=1 if filter present	−24.5*	−5.10*	−19.4*	−0.530*	−25.9*	−6.14*	−19.7*	−0.351
	(6.97)	(3.08)	(6.05)	(0.408)	(9.42)	(4.16)	(8.58)	(0.589)
Overall time trend	−1.32*	−1.10*	0.219	0.070*	No	No	No	No
	(0.836)	(0.369)	(0.725)	(0.049)				
Year dummies	Yes	Yes	Yes	Yes	Yes	Yes	Yes	Yes
City dummies	Yes	Yes	Yes	Yes	Yes	Yes	Yes	Yes
City-specific time trends	No	No	No	No	Yes	Yes	Yes	Yes
City-specific "waves"	No	No	No	No	Yes	Yes	Yes	Yes
No. of observations	190	190	190	190	190	190	190	190
Adjusted R^2	0.634	0.756	0.381	0.216	0.697	0.798	0.434	0.280

Source: See text.
Notes: Standard errors are reported in parentheses. An asterisk indicates significant at the 10 percent level or higher, one-tailed test. Variables are as defined in table 6.2.

Table 7.7
Race, Typhoid, and Filtration in Segregated Cities: Further Tests

	Segregated cities, with single time trend				Segregated cities, with city-specific "waves"			
	1a	1b	1c	1d	2a	2b	2c	2d
Variable	y^b	y^w	$y^b - y^w$	y^b/y^w	y^b	y^w	$y^b - y^w$	y^b/y^w
=1 if filter present	−7.30* (4.63)	−0.029 (3.50)	−7.27* (4.14)	0.033 (0.256)	−7.43* (5.70)	−4.56 (4.42)	−2.87 (5.47)	−0.031 (0.345)
Overall time trend	−2.57* (0.589)	−2.93* (0.445)	0.358 (0.526)	0.086* (0.033)	No	No	No	No
Year dummies	Yes	Yes	Yes	Yes	Yes	Yes	Yes	Yes
City dummies	Yes	Yes	Yes	Yes	Yes	Yes	Yes	Yes
City-specific time trends	No	No	No	No	Yes	Yes	Yes	Yes
City-specific "waves"	No	No	No	No	Yes	Yes	Yes	Yes
No. of observations	206	206	206	206	206	206	206	206
Adjusted R^2	0.580	0.647	0.249	0.138	0.683	0.720	0.348	0.223

Source: See text.
Notes: Standard errors are reported in parentheses. An asterisk indicates significant at the 10 percent level or higher, one-tailed test. Variables are as defined in table 6.2.

benefitted whites but not blacks. This suggests that disparities between black and white waterborne disease rates would have grown larger following improvements in water and sewer systems.

There are two ways to measure disparities in disease rates; one can examine either the ratio of, or the difference between, black and white rates. In chapter 6, both metrics were used. My goal in this section is to show that the choice of metric can matter, a possibility that was only alluded to in the previous chapter. To put things more sharply, in searching for evidence that the installation of water filters affected blacks and whites differently, the findings can change, depending on whether one uses the ratio of, or the difference between, disease rates for blacks and whites. In developing this point, I leave open, for the time being at least, questions about why these two metrics yield conflicting results, and questions about which metric provides the better indicator of unequal access. These questions are addressed in section 7.4.

Previous Efforts to Use Interracial Disparities in Disease Rates

Historians frequently use interracial disparities in disease rates as evidence of discrimination on the part of local officials and health providers. The rationale for using these rates is that it is difficult to observe the distribution of public health services directly. For example, there are only a handful of studies that were able to directly observe differences in the rates at which black and white households connected to public water and sewer lines in turn-of-the-century America. And in the case of these facilities, the data that are available cover only four cities, which are located largely in the South (see discussion in chapters 3 and 4). Unable to observe distributional differences in public health facilities directly, historians have been forced to turn to more easily accessible proxies, such as disease rates. (Chapters 3 and 4, however, present work in which I have been able to observe distributional differences directly.)

In the least satisfactory historical studies, the authors use cross-sectional data to document interracial differences in disease and death rates, and then argue that these differences reflect discrimination on the part of public health providers.[5] The difficulties with such crude comparisons are manifold. First, as is sometimes acknowledged, there are many potential causes for differences in disease rates across racial groups. To the extent that diet, age, marital status, exercise, housing conditions, employment, and occupation differ systematically across racial groups and these differences affect health, they would also generate racial disparities in disease rates. Clearly, there needs to be some effort to control for, and ultimately quantify, the relative importance of the various determinants of disease across racial groups before concluding that there was discrimination in the provision of public health. Second, with cross-sectional data, it will usually be impossible to control directly for any unobserved heterogeneity across racial groups. Genetic predispositions for particular diseases, or cultural habits that leave one group prone to disease, cannot be adequately controlled for without access to near-perfect knowledge. The simplest way to control for such unobserved heterogeneity is to employ panel data analysis, which allows the researcher to mimic a full information world and "dummy out" all (fixed) unobserved differences.

Not all historical studies employ uncontrolled, cross-sectional comparisons in their analysis of interracial disparities in disease rates. One exception in this regard is *New Men, New Cities, New South* by Don H. Doyle. Employing time series data, Doyle shows that in Nashville, Tennessee, the ratio of black to white death rates was positively correlated with public health expenditures; as the city spent more on its water and sewer system and other public health measures, white death rates fell more, in percentage terms, than black rates. Even during the Progressive Era (1900–1914), when public health systems experienced their most rapid and presumably most equitable expansion, Doyle finds evidence that the ratio of black to white death rates continued to rise. Based on this, he concludes that officials in Nashville channeled resources toward improving the health of whites; blacks were given secondary attention. Doyle, however, emphasizes that while black health could take a back seat to white health, it could not be "entirely neglected," because white officials saw blacks "as dangerous carriers of color-blind germs." Fear of epidemic diseases spreading from blacks to whites also might have played a role in promoting efforts to segregate the races in Nashville and other southern cities.[6]

Doyle's analysis suggests four avenues that are in need of further research and discussion. First, it remains to be seen if Nashville is representative of a larger historical experience. Second, it is not clear how to best measure discrimination in the provision of public health services, particularly water and sewer lines. Doyle focuses exclusively on the ratio of black to white death rates to identify disparities in treatment, but as explained later, other measures of discrimination (such as differences in disease rates) can yield conflicting results. Nor is it clear that overall death rates are the best indicators of the effectiveness of public health measures. If one examines black and white death rates in Nashville independently, neither appeared to fall after public health measures were introduced.[7] More revealing indicators of discrimination might be death rates from diseases that are likely to respond to public health measures, such as tuberculosis and typhoid fever.

Third, it would be useful to identify discrete and permanent changes in health policy, such as the installation of a water filter or the introduction of chlorination, and explore how disease rates were affected by such changes. The installation of a water filter typically had a large and immediate effect on waterborne disease rates, and hence such an event allows cleaner and more precise tests of disproportionate effects across racial groups.

Disease and Discrimination in Washington

To illustrate how the choice of metric matters, consider again the experience of Washington. Recall that the city installed water filters in 1906 and 1911, and began chlorinating its water supply in 1918. If African Americans had relatively limited access to the public water supply, these improvements would have benefitted only whites, or at least would have benefitted whites disproportionately. This suggests that the disparity between black and white typhoid rates in the city would have risen following the introduction of filtration and chlorination. To test this proposition, I examined the difference between, and the ratio of, black and white typhoid death rates.

Figure 7.4 plots this difference. It suggests that blacks, not whites, benefitted disproportionately from the installation of the first water filter. Before 1906, the difference between typhoid death rates for blacks and those for whites was as high as 65 points; between 1906 and 1911, it never rose above 20 points, one-third the size of the pre-1906 peak. The installation of the second water filter in 1911 appears to have benefitted whites slightly more since the difference in the rates rose to as high as 30 points, although this is still much lower than the gap that existed prior to 1906. The introduction of chlorination in 1918 had a dramatic and beneficial effect, reducing the difference between black and white typhoid death rates so that it hovered around 0 between 1919 and 1925. Overall, these patterns suggest that water purification benefitted blacks more than whites.

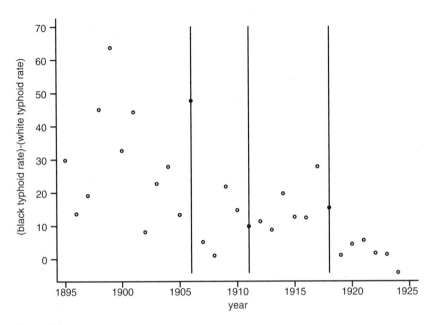

Figure 7.4
Difference between black and white typhoid death rates in Washington, D.C., 1895–1925.
Sources: U.S. Bureau of Census, *Mortality Statistics*, various years; U.S. Public Health Service, *Annual Reports*, various years.

However, a less optimistic interpretation is suggested by figure 7.5, which plots the ratio of black and white typhoid death rates. The ratio remained fairly constant after the installation of the first filter and rose sharply after the installation of the second filter. More precisely, after 1911, the ratio rose to historically unprecedented levels, so that black disease rates were as much as seven times greater than those for whites. Sustained improvement does not appear to have taken place until the introduction of chlorination in 1918, when the ratio fell from about 2 to less than 1. In short, the behavior of the ratio over time suggests that large relative improvements in black disease rates did not occur until 1920, about 15 years after the difference suggests that relative improvement first occurred.

7.4 Modeling Interracial Disparities: Choosing between Ratios and Levels

As explained earlier, recent historical works employ two alternative metrics to measure interracial disparities in disease rates. Some studies

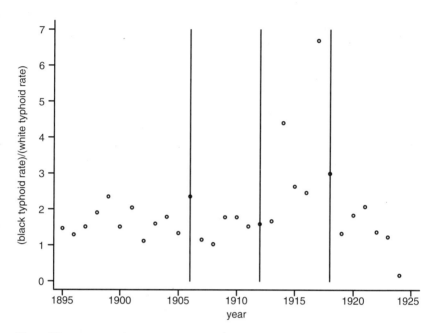

Figure 7.5
Ratio of black and white typhoid death rates in Washington, D.C., 1895–1925. Sources:
U.S. Bureau of Census, *Mortality Statistics*, various years and U.S. Public Health Service,
Annual Reports, various years.

use the ratio of black to white disease rates, while others use the difference between black and white rates.[8] The case study of Washington suggests that the choice of metric—ratio or difference—can be
determinative; ratios can yield one answer while differences can yield
another. Nevertheless, existing studies make no effort to justify the
decision to use one metric or the other, or to explore the robustness of
their findings to changes in the metric.

In this section I develop a formal model of the relationship between
typhoid death rates and water purity. Building a formal model allows
me to be precise about the assumptions behind using either the ratio
of, or the difference between, black and white mortality rates, and to
explore their usefulness in different contexts. Two key findings emerge
from the construction of the model. First, as an indirect measure of
access to health care, ratios and differences will only identify discrimination in worlds where discrimination is extreme. Where racial
disparities in access are slight, ratios and differences will have only
limited usefulness. Second, the preferability of one metric over another

depends on the time span the underlying data cover. When the data are truly long run, extending 30 years or more, the ratio is the preferred measure; when the data cover shorter periods of time, the difference is the preferred measure.

After constructing a formal model and identifying the assumptions that underlie it, I perform an empirical analysis of the parameters of the model. This analysis helps identify which metric—the ratio or the difference—is appropriate. More important, it suggests that the assumptions underlying the empirical work in chapter 6 are appropriate.

The Model

The following equations relate water quality to typhoid death rates for blacks (b) and whites (w) in a given city:

$$y^b = \alpha^b + \beta^b q \tag{7.1}$$

$$y^w = \alpha^w + \beta^w q, \tag{7.2}$$

where y^b and y^w are black and white typhoid death rates, respectively, and q is an inverse measure of the purity of the water distributed through public water mains so that increases in q imply reductions in water purity. By assumption, $q \in [0, \infty)$. Think of q as representing the number of bacteria contained in a unit of water, a common measure of water quality employed by public health officials in turn-of-the-century America. Because typhoid rates can never be negative and are always a positive function of q (as the number of bacteria in the water rises, disease rates also rise): $\alpha^k \geq 0$, and $\beta^k > 0$, $k = b, w$. The intercept α describes the level of typhoid that would prevail in a city where water from the public system is 100 percent free of bacteria. In such a city, typhoid would occur only when individuals not connected to the public system drew their water from impure sources, or more rarely, were exposed to other sources of infection such as tainted milk, flies, or shellfish from polluted rivers. The slope β describes how responsive black or white typhoid rates are to changes in the quality of the water distributed through the public system.[9]

In turn, both α and β are functions of various social, economic, demographic, and biological characteristics, so that:

$$\alpha^k = a(n^k, \mathbf{X}^k), \quad \text{and} \tag{7.3}$$

$$\beta^k = b(n^k, \mathbf{X}^k), \tag{7.4}$$

where $k = b$ or w; n^k is the proportion of the black or white population in the city connected to the public water supply so that $n^k \in [0, 1]$, and $\mathbf{X}^k$ is a vector of other characteristics affecting α and β. By assumption, α is a negative function of the proportion of the population connected to the public water supply, while β is a positive function: $a_n < 0$ and $b_n > 0$. These assumptions have reasonable implications. The first $(a_n < 0)$ implies that even when the city distributes water that is germ free $(q = 0)$, the level of typhoid would vary inversely with the proportion of the population connected to public water lines. The second $(b_n > 0)$ implies that holding everything else constant, the larger the proportion of the population connected to the water system, the more responsive typhoid death rates would be to changes in the quality of water from that system.

Three Plausible Scenarios

As indicated earlier, historians of public health must use either differences in, or ratios of, disease rates as proxies for access to services they cannot observe directly. With the model just constructed, it is now possible to examine the reliability of these proxies in different circumstances. This can be done by constructing a simulated world where the values of n^b and n^w are known and then identifying the accuracy of ratios and differences in competing scenarios.

To illustrate, consider first a city where blacks and whites have equal access to public water lines so that $n^b = n^w$. Even though the same proportion of blacks and whites are connected to public water lines, α and/or β would still vary by race because the other determinants of α and β, such as income, sanitary practices, and literacy, differ across racial groups. Two possible scenarios for this city are constructed.

Scenario 1

In the first scenario, assume the following: $n^b = n^w$; $\alpha^b > \alpha^w$; and $\beta^b = \beta^w$. Figure 7.6 illustrates. Initially the city does not filter its water and provides water of quality q_0. Typhoid death rates for blacks and whites are y_0^b and y_0^w, respectively. After the city begins filtering the water supply, q falls from q_0 to q_1 and with the improvement in water quality, typhoid death rates for blacks and whites fall to y_1^b and y_1^w, respectively. If we examine how the ratio of black to white typhoid rates changes following the introduction of filtration, we would find

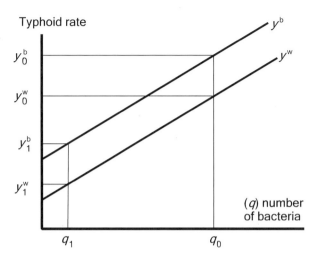

Figure 7.6
Typhoid and water quality, scenario 1. Source: See text.

evidence of discrimination; the ratio rises from $(y_0^b)/(y_0^w)$ to $(y_1^b)/(y_1^w)$.
To see that

$$(y_0^b)/(y_0^w) < (y_1^b)/(y_1^w), \tag{7.5}$$

note that with some minor algebraic manipulation we can rewrite expression (7.5) as

$$[(\alpha^b - \alpha^w)/(y_0^w)] < [(\alpha^b - \alpha^w)/(y_1^w)], \tag{7.6}$$

and we know by assumption that $y_0^w > y_1^w$. Alternatively, if instead of the ratio, we examine how the difference between black and white typhoid death rates changes after filtration, we would find evidence of equitable access to public water supplies; at both q_0 to q_1, the difference between black and white rates is $(\alpha^b - \alpha^w)$. In this case, the difference yields the correct answer, while the ratio is misleading.

Scenario 2
In the second scenario, assume the following: $n^b = n^w$; $\alpha^b = \alpha^w = 0$; and $\beta^b > \beta^w$. Figure 7.7 illustrates. We then proceed with the same experiment as in the first scenario. Initially the city does not filter its water and provides water of quality q_0. Typhoid death rates for blacks and whites are y_0^b and y_0^w, respectively. After the city begins filtering the water supply, q falls from q_0 to q_1, and with the improvement in

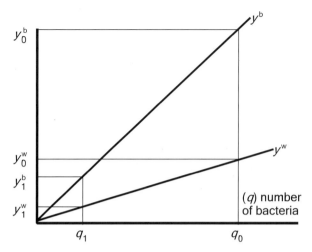

Figure 7.7
Typhoid and water quality, scenario 2. Source: See text.

water quality, typhoid death rates for blacks and whites fall to y_1^b and y_1^w. In this scenario, if we examine how the ratio of black to white typhoid rates changes following the introduction of filtration, we would find evidence of equitable access to public water supplies; at both q_0 and q_1, the ratio of black to white rates is $(\beta^b)/(\beta^w)$. Alternatively, if instead of the ratio we examine how the difference between black and white rates changes after filtration, we would find evidence that blacks benefitted more than whites from filtration, even though both groups had equal access to public water lines. To see that,

$$(y_1^b) - (y_1^w) < (y_0^b) - (y_0^w),\tag{7.7}$$

note that with some minor algebraic manipulation we can rewrite expression (7.7) as

$$(q_1) \times (\beta^b - \beta^w) < (q_0) \times (\beta^b - \beta^w),\tag{7.8}$$

and we know by assumption that $q_1 < q_0$. In this case, the ratio yields the correct answer while the difference is misleading.

Lessons from Scenarios 1 and 2
At this point, we should ask if either of these two scenarios provides a reasonable approximation of the true relationship between water quality and deaths from typhoid fever. While the next section uses historical data from North Carolina to formally estimate the parameters of

this model, it is useful to think about the answer to this question heuristically. Common sense and casual empiricism suggest that in the long run, say 20 or 30 years, the second scenario is a reasonable first-order approximation of the real world. Specifically, over the long haul, $\alpha^b = \alpha^w = 0$ and $\beta^b > \beta^w$, as long as blacks and whites have roughly similar proportions of their populations connected to public water lines (i.e., $n^b = n^w$). From two sources of evidence we know that $\beta^b > \beta^w$ when $n^b = n^w$. First, the qualitative evidence presented in chapter 3 suggests that whites were in a better position to fend off typhoid through private means and second, the empirical work discussed later suggests that even when $n^b < n^w$, that $\beta^b > \beta^w$. We know that $\alpha^b = \alpha^w = 0$ when $n^b = n^w = 1.00$ because once cities in the United States cleaned up their water supplies and connected all of their residents to public water systems, it was only a matter of time before typhoid disappeared. The only cases of typhoid that occur in the developed world today occur among citizens traveling to underdeveloped countries. Clearly, if $q = 0$ and $n = 1.0$ for a sufficient period of time, typhoid is a disease that will gradually disappear.

In the short run, however, in turn-of-the century America, even after all households were connected to public systems and public water was free of disease, typhoid remained endemic and could be spread through various forms of direct human contact and transmission, such as food handlers failing to properly wash their hands. As evidence for this, consider that in 1915, the two largest cities, New York and Chicago, both had nearly 100 percent of their populations connected to public water systems, and both cities chlorinated and/or filtered their water so that it was as free of disease-causing bacteria as water from public systems today. Yet in both cities, typhoid rates remained positive 5 or more years after the purification systems had been completed.

Together, scenarios 1 and 2 suggest an important caveat to the empirical work presented in chapter 6. Specifically, there are conditions under which the use of either ratios or differences will lead one to conclude there is no discrimination in provision of public water supplies, when in fact there is. To see this, note that $n^b < n^w$ does not necessarily imply that $\beta^b < \beta^w$, and as a result it is theoretically possible that variation in water quality from public water systems can affect blacks disproportionately despite the fact that there are proportionately fewer blacks connected to these systems. While it is difficult to say with any precision how plausible such contingencies are, it seems highly unlikely that they would occur in a world where the differences between

n^b and n^w are large. Indeed, in a city where there is extensive discrimination between black and white communities, either ratios or differences in disease rates would probably correctly identify the presence of inequitable access to service. A third scenario is constructed to illustrate this last point.

Scenario 3
Consider a city where discrimination is implemented perfectly; no African-American households are connected to public water lines, while all white households are. In terms of the model, $n^b = 0.0$ and $n^w = 1.0$. In such a city, it would be reasonable to assume that variation in the quality of water from the public system would affect white disease rates but have no effect on black rates because blacks were not connected to the water system: $\beta^b = 0$, $\beta^w > 0$. By the same token, black death rates would be high regardless of water quality, while those for whites would be very close to zero when water was bacteria free: $\alpha^b > 0$, $\alpha^w = 0$.

Figure 7.8 illustrates. Initially, water quality is imperfect and $q = q_0$. If public officials decide to improve water quality and begin filtering the public water supply, q falls from q_0 to q_1. White disease rates fall sharply following the improvement in water quality because 100 percent of white households are connected to the water system, while black rates do not fall because no black households are connected. Clearly, in a city where the relationship between disease and water

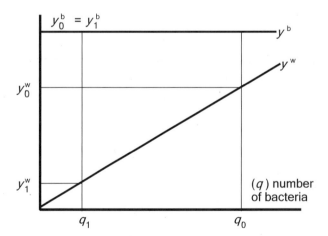

Figure 7.8
Typhoid and water quality, scenario 3. Source: See text.

quality is defined by parameters such as these, an increase in water quality (or a reduction in q) would cause both the ratio of, and the difference between, black and white typhoid death rates to rise.

Critical Assumptions and an Empirical Test

If disparities in disease rates are to help us draw reasonable inferences about the accessability of public water systems across racial groups, two previously stated assumptions are critical. First α^k must be a negative function of the proportion of the population connected to the public water supply and second, β^k must be a positive function. Stated in terms of the model described here, $a_n < 0$ and $b_n > 0$. If these conditions do not apply, disparities in disease rates can tell us nothing about discrimination in the public provision of water supplies. It is important to be clear that this is a general point and that it does not apply solely to the statistical work in this book. If these conditions do not hold, previous studies that use disparities in typhoid rates to draw inferences about discrimination in the provision of public facilities are also meaningless.[10]

To assess the validity of these two critical assumptions, data from turn-of-the-century North Carolina are employed. Between 1896 and 1902, the North Carolina State Board of Health regularly sampled the water supplies of various municipalities in the state. State health officials then counted the number of bacteria contained in a cubic centimeter of water and reported the results of those counts in the biennial reports of the board of health. Along with bacteria counts, the board also reported waterborne disease rates, by race, for the cities and towns in question.[11] In terms of our model, these data make it possible to observe both y^k and q. The other variables needed to explore the relationship between water quality, disease, and access to public water relate to the proportion of the population connected to the public water system: n^b and n^w. While data on the exact proportions connected to local water supplies are not available, it is possible to get reasonably close using the *Manual of American Water Works* published in 1897, and U.S. Census data.

With these sources, one can calculate miles of water mains per capita in each of the towns on which there are data on disease and proliferation of bacteria. While they are not as precise a measure of the extensiveness of local water systems as the proportion of population connected, the miles of water mains per capita provides a reasonable first-order approximation. Indeed, estimates reported in chapter 8 suggest that both measures (i.e., proportion connected and miles of mains per capita) perform equally well in regressions that explore the effect of improvements in water systems on waterborne disease rates for blacks and whites.

Table 7.8 summarizes the data. The disease rates refer to deaths per 100,000 persons from two waterborne diseases: typhoid fever and diarrhea. Except for Henderson and Tarboro, the rates for blacks are higher than those for whites. Bacterial counts vary dramatically across cities, from a low of 6 in Tarboro to a high of 25,000 in Wilmington. Even within cities there can be large differences from year to year. For example, in Salisbury, bacterial counts are as low as 22 per cubic centimeter in one year and as high as 14,400 in another. Because bacterial counts can vary by such large magnitudes, the data are also transformed with natural logarithms. The miles of water mains per 1,000 persons varies from a low of 0.60 in Tarboro to a high of 3.74 in Durham. In the median city, miles of water mains per 1,000 persons would have been 1.44.

With the North Carolina data in hand, it is possible to answer the central question of whether increases in n^k reduced α^k and increased β^k so that disease rates became more responsive to changes in water quality as public water systems were extended. This question is answered by implementing a three-step procedure. First, disease rates are regressed against water quality in municipalities with extensive water systems. Second, the same regressions are then run for municipalities with limited systems. Third, the regression results are compared across municipalities with extensive and limited systems. A municipality is said to have had an extensive water system if the number for miles of water mains per capita in that city was greater than that for the median city. A municipality is said to have had a limited water system if the number for miles of water mains per capita was below the median. Run separately for each race as well as for municipalities with limited (below-median) and extensive (above-median) water systems, the regressions estimate the parameters of Eqs. (7.1) and (7.2). All regressions have been weighted by population to control for the fact that disease rates would have been measured with greater accuracy in large towns than in small ones. (Unweighted regressions yield very similar estimates.)

Table 7.9 contains the regression results. Although the data are noisy, changes in the point estimates of α (the constant) and β (the co-

Table 7.8
Bacterial Counts, Disease, and Access to Public Water in a Panel of North Carolina Towns

City	Miles of water mains per 1,000 persons	Years observed	Disease rate[a]		Bacteria per cm[b]			Natural log(bacteria)		
			Black	White	Mean	Min.	Max.	Mean	Min.	Max.
Asheville	1.02	1900, 1902	281.3	171.1	266	52	480	5.06	3.95	6.17
Charlotte	0.86	All[c]	307.2	248.3	274	80	600	5.34	4.38	6.40
Durham	3.74	1900, 1902	744.8	319.4	448	56	840	5.38	4.03	6.73
Fayetteville	2.97	1897, 1902	265.5	137.9	140	120	180	4.92	4.79	5.19
Goldsboro	1.45	1897, 1900, 1902	352.8	280.1	1,784	33	6,800	5.45	3.50	8.82
Greensboro	1.20	1896, 1897, 1902	398.7	178.4	1,258	150	3,400	6.19	5.01	8.13
Henderson	2.14	All[c]	300.0	473.9	4,331	184	16,000	6.84	5.21	9.68
Raleigh	2.13	1897, 1900, 1902	327.6	291.0	463	76	1,300	5.61	4.33	7.17
Salem	1.87	All[c]	459.9	130.4	513	120	1,200	5.89	4.79	7.09
Salisbury	1.43	All[c]	479.9	447.0	3,681	22	14,400	5.66	3.09	9.57
Tarboro	0.60	1900, 1902	45.8	215.5	783	6	1,560	4.57	1.79	7.35
Wilmington	0.70	1896, 1902	406.1	301.9	14,300	3,600	25,000	9.16	8.19	10.12
Wilson	1.77	1896, 1897, 1900	268.0	232.6	120	56	154	4.69	4.02	5.04
All cities	1.44 (median)	41 obs.	357.6	271.8	1,959.6	6	25,000	5.73	1.79	10.13

Sources: Baker, *Waterworks*, pp. 246–50; and North Carolina State Board of Health, *Biennial Report*, 1896–1902.
[a] White (or black) disease rate is measured as white (or black) deaths from waterborne diseases (diarrhea and typhoid) per 100,000 persons.
[b] The number of bacteria contained in a cubic centimeter of water from the public water system.
[c] "All" indicates the municipality has observations for all years from 1896 through 1902.

Table 7.9
Water Quality and Waterborne Disease Rates for Blacks and Whites

	White waterborne disease rate				Black waterborne disease rate					
	Limited water		Extensive water		Limited water		Extensive water			
Variable	1a	1b	2a	2b	3a	3b	4a	4b	4c	4d
ln(bacteria)[a]	16.8	30.0	46.9*	98.3*	14.7	26.5	77.0	53.1	133.7*	152.6*
	(14.6)	(23.2)	(23.1)	(29.7)	(14.8)	(24.7)	(53.8)	(70.6)	(65.0)	(93.1)
Constant[b]	160.2	150.9	10.6	−337.2*	261.8*	150.9	−60.1	257.0	−356.8	−382.6
	(94.3)	(154.8)	(132.0)	(182.6)	(95.8)	(247.8)	(307.1)	(433.9)	(360.0)	(537.1)
Year dummies	No	Yes	No	Yes	No	Yes	No	Yes	No	Yes
N	21	21	20	20	21	21	20	20	19	19
R^2	0.065	0.210	0.186	0.494	0.050	0.120	0.052	0.335	0.200	0.433

Source: See text.

Notes: Standard errors are reported in parentheses. An asterisk indicates significant at the 10 percent level or higher (one-tailed test). Disease rates are measured as deaths from waterborne diseases (diarrhea and typhoid) per 100,000 persons. "Limited water" towns are those with miles of water mains per 1,000 persons below the median city (1.44). "Extensive water" towns are those with miles of water per 1,000 persons above the median.
[a] The coefficient on the natural log of the bacteria count corresponds to β in the formal model.
[b] The coefficient on the constant term corresponds to α in the formal model.

efficient on the natural log of the bacterial count) across limited and extensive cities are consistent with the assumption that disease rates grew more responsive to changes in water quality as water systems became more extensive. For whites in extensive cities, the estimates of β are about 3 times greater than the estimates of β in limited cities. Similarly, the estimates of α in extensive cities, depending upon specification, are about one-tenth to one-third the size of the estimates for limited cities. For blacks there are also pronounced differences across extensive and limited cities, although the data for blacks are even noisier than those for whites and are sensitive to the treatment of one outlying observation—the town of Henderson in 1902. If the outlier is included, the estimates of β in extensive cities are 1.5 to 5 times greater than in limited cities, and in one specification α is much smaller in extensive cities than in limited ones. Compare regressions 3a and 3b with regressions 4a and 4b. If the outlier is dropped, the contrast between municipalities with extensive and limited water systems is even starker.

Figures 7.9 and 7.10 illustrate the differences in parameter estimates across municipalities with extensive and limited water systems. For whites, the estimates from regressions 1a and 2a are used. For blacks, the estimates from regressions 3a and 4a are used. The patterns depicted here provide strong support for the idea that variation in water quality had a larger effect on disease rates in towns with relatively extensive water systems than in those with limited systems. The results also suggest two important implications. First, variation in water quality appears to have had a larger impact on black disease rates than on white rates. As shown in chapter 3, the most plausible explanation for this finding is that African-American households were less able than white households to engage in the personal precautions necessary to prevent typhoid. Second, the fact that extensions in water systems made black disease rates more responsive to variation in water quality suggests that when cities built new water lines, they were not installing them solely in white neighborhoods.

Key Findings

This section has built a formal model relating waterborne disease rates to water quality. The model suggests that in a world where there are extreme racial disparities in access to public water lines, the use of either differences in, or ratios of, disease rates will yield accurate

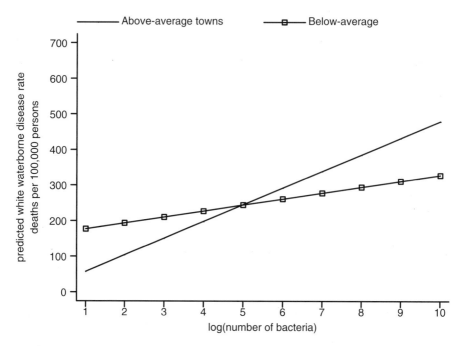

Figure 7.9
Water quality, typhoid, and access to public water: relationships for whites. Above-average towns are those with extensive water systems. The plots show the relationship between water quality (q) and the waterborne disease rate for whites. Below-average towns have relatively limited water systems and the plots show the relationship between water quality and waterborne disease rates for whites. Source: See text.

conclusions about the presence of discrimination. If, however, racial disparities in access to public water lines are slight, differences and ratios might yield conflicting results, and the choice of metric would depend on the underlying data. In particular, if the underlying data are truly long run, covering, say, 30 years, the ratio of disease rates would be appropriate. On the other hand, if the data cover only a short time horizon, say 10–20 years, the difference between black and white disease rates would probably be the better way to identify inequalities in access to public water lines.

This section has also identified two key assumptions that must hold if racial disparities in waterborne disease rates are to tell us anything meaningful about discrimination in the provision of public water supplies. More precisely, for disparities in disease to tell us something meaningful, it must be the case that as the proportion of the population connected to public water lines increases, waterborne disease rates be-

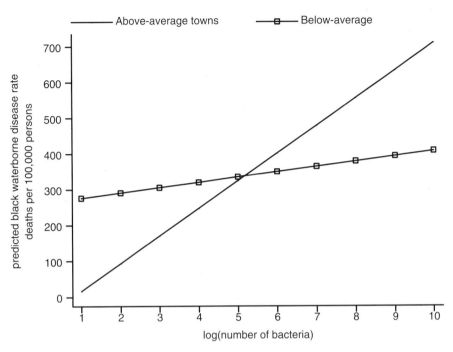

Figure 7.10
Water quality, typhoid, and access to public water: relationships for blacks. Above-average towns have extensive water systems. The plots show the relationship between water quality (q) and waterborne disease rates for blacks. Below-average towns have relatively limited water systems and the plots show relationship between water quality and waterborne disease rates for blacks. Source: See text.

come more responsive to changes in the quality of the water from public supplies. The data from North Carolina suggest that these key assumptions hold. In North Carolina municipalities with relatively extensive water systems, variation in water quality had a much larger effect on waterborne disease rates than in municipalities with limited water systems.

7.5   Are the Data on Typhoid Mortality Reliable?

In previous chapters I relied heavily on data on mortality rates. In this section I discuss two concerns associated with using data on typhoid mortality. The first involves the preferability of using incidence rates. I argue that while data on incidence rates are often preferable to data on mortality, with typhoid the distinction between incidence and mortality data is unimportant. Both will yield similar answers, largely because there were no effective clinical treatments for the disease before 1940. The second concern focuses on the fact that typhoid was sometimes mistakenly diagnosed as malaria. After constructing a hypothetical example to illustrate the implications of typhoid undercounts, case studies of two cities—Jacksonville and Richmond—are presented. Based on the case studies, I argue that blacks were much more likely to have had typhoid mistakenly diagnosed as malaria than were whites. I also argue that the failure to control for the tendency to confuse typhoid with malaria biases the econometric work in chapter 6 against finding evidence that filtration benefitted blacks disproportionately.

Incidence versus Mortality Rates

One might argue that data on incidence rates would be preferable to my data on mortality rates. To see this, recall the preceding discussion about water filtration in Washington. These data appear to show deaths from typhoid fever falling after the installation of water filters in 1906 and 1911. The case for filtration causing these reductions would be clarified if, rather than knowing how many people died of typhoid, we knew how many people actually contracted the disease. This is because the number of deaths could have been determined not only by water quality but also by the quality of medical care received by those suffering from typhoid. If the quality of medical care improved over time, the data on death rates would conflate the effects of improved medical care with the effects of improved water quality. Moreover, given the focus here on racial disparities in mortality rates, there is a concern that access to effective medical treatments might have differed across racial groups.

Not surprisingly, there is evidence that whites had access to better medical care and treatment. Consider the experience of Jacksonville, where between 1908 and 1911 there was no attending physician in 17 percent of all African-American deaths, while in contrast there was no attending physician in only 5 percent of all white deaths.[12] It is not likely, however, that this would have made any difference in treating typhoid. As explained in chapter 2, there were no effective clinical treatments for this disease before the introduction of antibiotics in the 1940s. All doctors could do for typhoid sufferers in 1910 was recommend rest and a healthy diet. Given the absence of effective clinical treatments before the 1940s, it seems highly unlikely that quality of physician care could have affected the probability of surviving typhoid before this period. It might have affected the accuracy of the diagnosis, but that is another matter, which is discussed in the following section.

Confusing Typhoid and Malaria: Implications for Analysis of Data

Another concern is that typhoid was sometimes underreported and that this underreporting was reduced over time as the disease and its causes became better understood. As explained in chapter 2, deaths from typhoid were often mistakenly reported as deaths from malaria. There are two ways to address the concern that underreporting of typhoid was reduced over time. The first is to estimate true typhoid rates and adjust the reported rates accordingly. One simple approach along these lines would be to add malaria and typhoid rates together and explore their joint behavior. If there were no secular trends in malaria rates, either downward or upward, this procedure would provide a reasonable way to assess changes in typhoid rates over time.

The second way to address this concern is to think precisely about what biases have been introduced into the data, and about how those biases affect our interpretations. In this regard, the trend away from underreporting suggests that if we plot (observed) typhoid rates over time, we will understate the true reduction in typhoid death rates that occurred between, say, 1880 and 1920. This in turn suggests that all tests involving time-series data will be biased against finding beneficial effects of water filtration in the absence of any adjustments to the underlying data. To the extent that African Americans benefitted disproportionately from improvements in water systems, this means that the tests will also understate the magnitude of these (disproportionate) benefits.

To see this, consider figure 7.11, which plots observed and actual typhoid rates for a hypothetical city over time. The observed typhoid rates (y^O) are those reported by public officials, and these observed rates may or may not equal actual typhoid rates (y^A). Whether observed and actual rates converge depends on the accuracy of the diagnosis of the attending physician. To keep the discussion simple, there is one critical date, t^*. At t^*, doctors discover what causes typhoid and are therefore able to diagnose the disease perfectly. So after t^*, observed and actual typhoid rates are equal: $y^O = y^A$. But before t^*, typhoid is poorly understood and doctors are reluctant to diagnose it. As a result, some fraction of all deaths from typhoid are mistakenly reported as deaths from malaria, and observed typhoid rates are much less than actual rates: $y^O < y^A$.

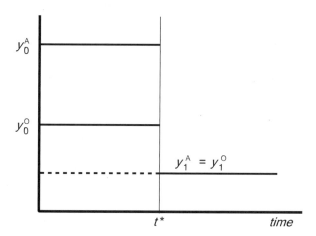

Figure 7.11
Estimated benefits of filtration with typhoid undercounts. Source: See text.

However, t^* is important, not just because it is the date that doctors discover how to properly diagnose typhoid, it is also important because the same scientific discoveries that facilitate proper diagnosis also facilitate the design of effective public health measures to combat typhoid, such as the installation of water filters. The scientific discovery implied here is the formulation of the germ theory of disease, which as explained earlier, was instrumental in helping devise effective strategies for diagnosing and preventing typhoid fever. So the hypothetical city installs a water filter at t^*. Suppose now that we want to measure the benefits of filtration for this hypothetical city. If we use observed typhoid rates, the estimated benefits of filtration, in terms of disease reduction, would be $y_0^O - y_1^O$. Yet the actual benefits of filtration would be $y_0^A - y_1^A$. Because $y_0^A > y_0^O$, and $y_1^A = y_1^O$, $[y_0^A - y_1^A] > [y_0^O - y_1^O]$. This suggests that in the absence of adjusting for the underreporting of typhoid during the late nineteenth and very early twentieth centuries, estimates of the benefits of water filtration would be biased downward.

Typhoid and Typhomalaria in Jacksonville and Richmond

To illustrate the effects of the underreporting of typhoid fever more concretely, consider the experiences of Jacksonville and Richmond. As explained in chapter 4, Jacksonville had a serious problem with typhoid fever, and only implemented measures to combat that problem

Table 7.10
Malaria, Typhoid, and Typhomalaria in Jacksonville

Disease	Average death rate per 100,000 persons		Absolute reduction	Percent reduction
	1906–1911	1912–1917		
Black typhoid fever rate	82.7	21.4	61.3	0.74
Black malaria rate	101.5	16.9	84.6	0.83
Black typhoid fever rate + black malaria rate	184.2	38.3	146.0	0.79
White typhoid fever rate	113.5	33.1	80.5	0.71
White malaria rate	25.0	6.6	18.4	0.74
White typhoid fever rate + white malaria rate	138.5	39.7	98.8	0.71

Sources: U.S. Bureau of Census, *General Statistics of Cities*, 1915 and *Mortality Statistics*, various years; Terry, "The Negro."

in 1911. Table 7.10 summarizes typhoid and malaria rates for blacks and whites in this city. Data are provided for before and after 1911, the year the antityphoid measures were implemented.

Two patterns suggest that among blacks in Jacksonville, typhoid was frequently mistaken for malaria. First, notice that typhoid rates for blacks seem implausibly low compared with rates for whites. During the 1906–1911 period, black typhoid rates were, on average, 27 percent lower than those for whites; during the 1912–1917 period, they were 35.3 percent lower. By the same token, malaria rates for blacks seem implausibly high. It is well known that persons of African descent have a higher level of genetic resistance to malaria than Europeans. This heightened level of resistance is related to black vulnerability to sickle-cell anemia; sickle-shaped red blood cells are relatively inhospitable hosts for the malarial plasmodium.[13] Yet malaria rates for blacks in Jacksonville are four times greater than malaria rates for whites. It is odd that typhoid—a disease that is highly correlated with poverty and poor sanitation—should be less common among blacks than whites, while at the same time malaria—a disease that is spread by a mosquito and a disease for which blacks have an innate resistance—would be much more common among blacks than whites.[14]

The second suggestive pattern relates to the responsiveness of malaria rates to measures designed to prevent typhoid. There is no reason why filtering water and screening privies, both of which were aimed at combating typhoid in Jacksonville, should have reduced malaria rates in the city. Yet, for both blacks and whites, malaria rates plummeted following the implementation of antityphoid measures in 1911: black malaria rates fell by 83 percent and those for whites by 74 percent (see table 7.10). In contrast, typhoid rates also fell, but by a smaller amount; black typhoid rates fell by 74 percent after 1911 and rates for whites fell by 71 percent.

A likely explanation for the mysteriously low typhoid rates among blacks is that cases of typhoid in this group were mistakenly diagnosed as cases of malaria. The data on typhoid mortality certainly appear more reasonable if black typhoid rates are adjusted by adding the black malaria rate to the black typhoid rate. During the 1906–1911 period, black typhomalaria rates exceed white typhoid rates by 63 percent, and white typhomalaria rates by 33 percent. During the 1912–1919 period, black typhomalaria rates exceed white typhoid rates by 15 percent, and white typhomalaria rates by −3.5 percent. Notice that the estimated benefits of the antityphoid measures of 1911 are lower if no effort is made to adjust black typhoid rates; without any adjustment, black rates fall by 61.3 points (74 percent) after 1911; with the crude malaria adjustment, black rates fall by 146 points (79 percent).[15]

The identical findings emerge when disease rates in Richmond are analyzed. Figure 7.12 plots the typhoid rates for blacks and whites observed from 1900 through 1920. Vertical lines in the figure indicate the installation of a water filtration system in 1909 and the introduction of chlorination in 1917. In the prefiltration era, 1900–1908, black typhoid rates appear implausibly low; in 6 of the 9 years, white typhoid rates are greater than black rates and, on average, they exceed black rates by 12 percent. During this same time, public health officials in Richmond observed that the reported malaria rates in the city struck them as too high. They believed that inaccurate diagnoses by a few doctors in the city inflated these rates. And indeed, of the 200 doctors who practiced medicine in Richmond, three were responsible for 69 percent of all deaths reported as resulting from malaria, while other doctors with much larger practices typically reported no more than one death a year from malaria. Put another way, these three doctors (individually) were 146 times more likely than the average Richmond doctor to have reported a patient dying from malaria.[16]

Table 7.11 provides further evidence that typhoid was being mistaken for malaria in Richmond, particularly among blacks. As the table shows, black malaria rates averaged 43 deaths per 100,000 persons during the prefiltration era, while white malaria rates averaged only 7.

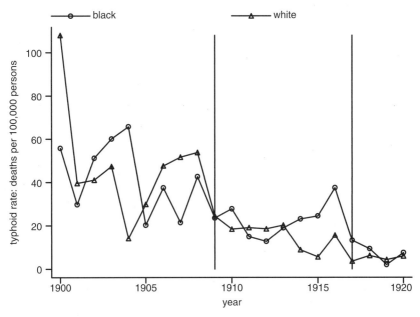

Figure 7.12
Observed typhoid fever rates in Richmond, 1900–1920. Vertical lines indicate the instal-
lation of a water filter in 1909 and the introduction of chlorination around 1917. Sources:
U.S. Bureau of Census, *General Statistics of Cities*, 1915 (data prepared by Center for Pop-
ulation Economics); *American City* (no author), "Water Supply Statistics"; U.S. Bureau of
Census, *Mortality Statistics*, various years and *Census*, 1900; Hoffman, "Progressive Public
Health."

As in Jacksonville, this disparity is surprising and suggestive. Blacks
were six times more likely than whites to have died of malaria, yet
blacks were *less* likely than whites to have died of typhoid. As explained earlier, this is surprising because typhoid was a disease that
was highly correlated with poverty and poor sanitation, while malaria
was a disease for which blacks had an innate resistance. Clearly something was amiss.[17]

If one fails to control for doctors misdiagnosing typhoid as malaria,
improvements in water quality in Richmond appear to have benefitted
whites disproportionately, although both blacks and whites benefitted
to some degree. This can be seen in table 7.11. For blacks, the death
rate from typhoid in the prefiltration era averaged 43 deaths per
100,000 persons and for whites it was 48; while during the filtration era
the death rate for blacks averaged 18 and that for whites 13 per 100,000
persons, a reduction of 58 and 70 percent, respectively. However, if

Table 7.11
Malaria, Typhoid, and Typhomalaria in Richmond

Disease	Average death rate per 100,000 persons		Absolute reduction	Percent reduction
	1900–1908	1909–1920		
Black typhoid fever rate	42.7	17.9	24.8	0.581
Black malaria rate	43.1	2.1	41.0	0.953
Black typhoid fever rate + black malaria rate	85.8	20.0	65.8	0.767
White typhoid fever rate	48.1	12.6	35.5	0.738
White malaria rate	7.0	1.8	5.2	0.743
White typhoid fever rate + white malaria rate	55.1	14.4	40.7	0.739

Sources: U.S. Bureau of Census, *General Statistics of Cities*, 1915; *American City* (no author), "Water Supply Statistics"; U.S. Bureau of Census, *Mortality Statistics*, various years and *Census*, 1900; Hoffman, "Progressive Public Health."
Notes: Malaria rates by race are available for 1900 and 1906–1920. For 1901–1905, malaria rates for each race are inferred from overall malaria rates.

one controls for typhoid undercounts by combining typhoid and malaria rates, the evidence that whites benefitted disproportionately vanishes, and if anyone benefitted disproportionately, it appears to have been African Americans. For blacks, deaths from typhomalaria in the prefiltration era averaged 86 per 100,000 persons and for whites 55; while during the filtration era, the death rate for blacks averaged 20 and that for whites was 14, a reduction of 77 and 75 percent, respectively.

Figure 7.13 plots the difference between black and white typhoid rates, and that between black and white typhomalaria rates. This figure encapsulates the preceding discussion. It shows that in the prefiltration era, black victims of typhoid were more likely to have had their deaths erroneously attributed to malaria than were white victims. It also shows that if one uses observed typhoid rates rather than typhomalaria rates, this would understate the extent to which blacks gained, relative to whites, from water filtration and purification.[18]

Key Findings

This section has developed two arguments. First, because there were no effective clinical treatments for typhoid before 1940, the mortality

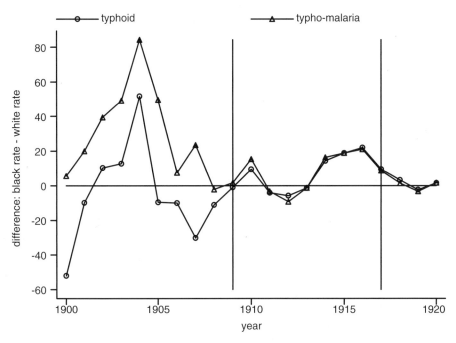

Figure 7.13
Black-white differences in typhoid and typhomalaria rates, 1900–1920. Vertical lines indicate the installation of a water filter in 1909 and the start of chlorination around 1917. Sources: U.S. Bureau of Census, *General Statistics of Cities*, 1915 (data prepared by Center for Population Economics); *American City*, "Water Supply Statistics"; U.S. Bureau of Census, *Mortality Statistics*, various years and *Census*, 1900; Hoffman, "Progressive Public Health."

data on typhoid used throughout this book yield answers that are very similar to those that would be obtained using data on the incidence of typhoid, which unfortunately are not available for the cities and time periods considered here. Second, in southern cities, deaths from typhoid were sometimes mistakenly attributed to malaria, and the tendency to confuse typhoid with malaria introduces a bias into the data. If the researcher ignores this bias, comparisons of typhoid rates before and after water filtration will understate the benefits of filtration, and more important, will understate the extent to which African Americans benefitted disproportionately from water filtration. This last result occurs in part because blacks were much more likely than whites to have had typhoid mistakenly diagnosed as malaria.[19]

7.5   Conclusions

Briefly, the key findings of this chapter are as follows: First, the findings in chapter 6 are robust to all reasonable respecifications in my
econometric model, and under many respecifications, the findings in
chapter 6 are strengthened. Second, the assumptions that underlie the
statistical analysis in chapter 6 receive strong support from independent sources of evidence, and the data used in chapter 6, while compromised, are compromised in a way that biases the results against my
larger argument. Based on the evidence in this chapter, I would argue
that, if anything, the findings in chapter 6 *understate* the extent to
which blacks benefitted disproportionately from investments in public
water filters.

8   Further Tests

8.1   Introduction

This chapter presents two additional sets of statistical tests. The first set explores the degree to which extensions in local water systems had disproportionate effects on black and white waterborne disease rates. The evidence of disproportionate effects is then used to draw inferences about the accessibility of water mains across racial groups. While the analysis thus far has used disease rates to isolate inequities in service, the second set of tests uses an alternative measure: city-wide growth in miles of water mains installed. The intuition that guides this analysis is straightforward. If cities were providing black neighborhoods with fewer water mains than white neighborhoods, city-wide growth in main mileage would have been less responsive to increases in the black population than it was to increases in the white population.[1]

8.2   Test One

Data and Estimation Strategy

For the first set of tests, waterborne disease rates are assembled by race for fifteen American cities in 1908. The rates are measured as deaths per 100,000 persons from diarrhea and typhoid fever. Including all cities for which data are available, the sample consists of the following cities: Wilmington, Delaware; Atlanta, Georgia; Savannah, Georgia; Baltimore, Maryland; Boston, Massachusetts; Kansas City, Missouri; St. Louis, Missouri; Cincinnati, Ohio; Philadelphia, Pennsylvania; Pittsburgh, Pennsylvania; Memphis, Tennessee; Nashville, Tennessee; Gal-

veston, Texas; Norfolk, Virginia; and Richmond, Virginia. Data on
waterborne disease rates are from the U.S. Bureau of the Census's
Mortality Statistics, and data on local water systems are from the
bureau's *General Statistics of Cities* and *The McGraw Directory of American Water Companies*.

With these data, variants on the following three equations are
estimated:

$$bwat = \alpha_b + \beta_b watcap + \delta_b btotdr + \lambda_b wat00 + \varepsilon_b \tag{8.1}$$

$$wwat = \alpha_w + \beta_w watcap + \delta_w wtotdr + \lambda_w wat00 + \varepsilon_w \tag{8.2}$$

$$diffwat = \alpha_d + \beta_d watcap + \delta_1 btotdr + \delta_2 wtotdr + \lambda_d wat00 + \varepsilon_d, \tag{8.3}$$

where *bwat* (*wwat*) is the black (or white) waterborne disease rate in
city *i* in 1908; *diffwat* is the difference between, or the ratio of, the black
and white waterborne disease rates; *watcap* equals miles of water
mains per 100,000 persons in city *i*; *btotdr* (*wtotdr*) is the overall black
(or white) death rate, measured as deaths per 100,000 persons from all
causes, except waterborne diseases; *wat00* is the overall waterborne
disease rate (i.e., the average disease rate across blacks and whites) in
city *i* in 1900; and the *ε*s are random-error terms. (Note that for the
moment the possibility of disease spillovers is ignored; this issue is
explored in the next section.)

Miles of water mains per 100,000 persons in 1908 (*watcap*) is a proxy
for the extensiveness of local water systems. To control for the possible
endogeneity between water mains per capita and disease rates, instrumental variables are employed. The ownership of local gas companies
(whether public or private) and miles of unimproved streets per acre of
land serve as instruments. As measures of the level of development in
public infrastructure, these variables would have been correlated with
miles of water mains per capita, but not disease rates. The inclusion of
total mortality rates (*btotdr* and *wtotdr*) controls for the overall health of
the black and white populations. The inclusion of overall waterborne
disease rates in 1900 (*wat00*) has an effect similar to that of including a
lag of the dependent variable. It controls for unobservable characteristics not otherwise accounted for. All regressions have been weighted
by black, white, or total population to control for the possibility that
disease rates were measured with greater accuracy in large cities than
in small ones.

The variable of primary interest is *watcap*. Consider four plausible
hypotheses and the coefficient estimates they imply.

Hypothesis 8.1

By 1908, cities had completed installing water mains in white neighborhoods and were extending service to black neighborhoods. In this case, variation in main mileage per capita would have been driven by differences in the level of water service available to black neighborhoods across cities. Consequently, in cities with relatively low main mileage per capita, black waterborne disease rates would have been higher, while white disease rates would have been unaffected. This implies the following coefficient estimates: $\beta_w = 0$, $\beta_b < 0$ and $\beta_d < 0$.

Hypothesis 8.2

In 1908, cities were installing water mains in white neighborhoods and were not installing mains in black neighborhoods. In this case, variation in main mileage per capita would have been driven by differences in the level of water service available to white neighborhoods across cities. Consequently, in cities with relatively low main mileage per capita, white waterborne disease rates would have been higher, while black rates would have been unaffected. This implies the following coefficient estimates: $\beta_w < 0$, $\beta_b = 0$, and $\beta_d > 0$.

Hypothesis 8.3

In 1908, cities were installing water mains in both black and white neighborhoods. In this case, a variation in main mileage per capita would have been driven by differences in the level of water service available to both neighborhoods across cities. Consequently, in cities with relatively low main mileage per capita, both black and white waterborne disease rates would have been higher. This implies the following coefficient estimates: $\beta_w = \beta_b \leq 0$, and $\beta_d = 0$.

Hypothesis 8.4

By 1908, cities had completed installing water mains in white neighborhoods and were not extending service to black neighborhoods. In this case, there would have been little variation in main mileage per capita, and whatever variation there was would have had little effect on either white or black disease rates. This implies the following coefficient estimates: $\beta_w = \beta_b = \beta_d = 0$.

Results and Supplemental Evidence

Table 8.1 contains the regression results, which contradict the idea embodied in hypotheses 8.2 and 8.4 that blacks had no access to urban

Table 8.1
Water Mains and Black and White Waterborne Disease Rates in Fifteen American Cities, 1908

Variable	Mean (S.D.)	OLS				2SLS			
		Black[a]	White[b]	Black − white[c]	Black/ white[c]	Black[a]	White[b]	Black − white[c]	Black/ white[c]
Black waterborne disease rate, 1908	216.0 (76.6)	Dep. var.	…	…	…	Dep. var.	…	…	…
White waterborne disease rate, 1908	151.9 (39.1)	…	Dep. var.	…	…	…	Dep. var.	…	…
Black − white	64.0 (78.0)	…	…	Dep. var.	…	…	…	Dep. var.	…
Black/white	1.48 (0.62)	…	…	…	Dep. var.	…	…	…	Dep. var.
Miles of water mains per 100,000 persons[d]	122.3 (16.7)	−3.56* (3.44)	−1.05* (3.63)	−2.75* (3.65)	−0.012* (2.69)	−4.00* (2.37)	−1.24* (3.65)	−3.17* (3.53)	−0.011* (2.35)
Black total death rate, except waterborne	2,461 (466)	0.049 (1.15)	…	0.104* (3.74)	0.001* (3.99)	0.045 (1.00)	…	0.106* (3.77)	0.001* (3.98)
White total death rate, except waterborne	1,485 (136)	…	0.118* (3.68)	−0.129 (1.48)	−0.001* (1.86)	…	0.114* (3.46)	−0.141 (1.57)	−0.001* (1.86)
Ave. waterborne disease rate, 1900	176.4 (47.8)	−0.025 (0.071)	0.643* (7.34)	−0.265 (1.07)	−0.256* (1.49)	−0.010 (0.03)	0.643* (7.20)	−0.266 (1.06)	−0.256 (1.49)
Constant	…	521.6* (2.70)	−13.8 (0.19)	374.1* (2.01)	3.36* (2.59)	580.8* (2.19)	14.8 (0.20)	433.7* (2.16)	3.41* (2.47)
No. of observations	15	15	15	15	15	15	15	15	15
Adjusted R^2		0.494	0.832	0.618	0.600	0.485	0.826	0.606	0.599

Sources: See text.
Notes: t-Statistics are in parentheses. An asterisk indicates significant at the 10 percent level (two-tailed test).
[a] Regression weighted by black population.
[b] Regression weighted by white population.
[c] Regression weighted by total population.
[d] In two-stage regressions, percentage of gas companies that were municipally owned in the state where the city was located, and miles of unimproved street per acre of land serve as instruments.

water systems as of 1908. Variation in main mileage per capita affected waterborne disease rates among blacks, suggesting that at least some black neighborhoods had access to public water supplies. This variation also reduced waterborne disease rates among whites, suggesting that in the cities where water systems were incomplete, it was not only blacks who were going without service. However, the results also show that increases in mileage per capita reduced the ratio of, and the difference between, black and white waterborne disease rates. This suggests that variation in main mileage affected blacks disproportionately and that blacks were the most likely to have gone without service when water systems were not complete.

As a check on the 1908 sample, which includes only fifteen cities, a second sample was assembled and analyzed. This sample included twenty-three American cities observed in 1911 (see table 8.2). Although the results are not quite as strong as those reported for 1908, the 1911 data point in the same general direction: Variation in main mileage per capita affected blacks disproportionately.

A concern with both the 1908 and 1911 regressions is that water mains per capita is an indirect measure of extensiveness of service. A more direct measure, such as the proportion of homes in the city connected to the system, would be desirable. To address this concern, data on waterborne disease rates by race as of 1915 were assembled for thirty-five American cities. The proportion of all homes connected to the local water system as of 1915 (percent connected) was used as a measure of access to service. Unfortunately, percent connected is an aggregate, city-wide measure and is not available by the racial makeup of homes; nor is it available for earlier years. To control for the potential endogeneity between typhoid rates and percent connected, instrumental variables were employed. The number of fire hydrants per capita and the tons of garbage collected per capita served as instruments. All regressions were weighted by black, white, or total population to control for the possibility that disease rates were measured with greater accuracy in large cities than in small ones.

The regression results in table 8.3 corroborate those obtained with the 1908 and 1911 data. Again, blacks were affected more by variation in levels of service than were whites, suggesting that when cities had water systems that did not reach the entire population, blacks were more likely than whites to have gone without service. Because variation in service levels had little impact on white disease rates, it would appear that by 1915 nearly all whites were enjoying service from local water companies.

Table 8.2
Water Mains and Black and White Waterborne Disease Rates in Twenty-Three American Cities, 1911

Variable	Mean (S.D.)	OLS Black[a]	OLS White[b]	OLS Black − white[c]	OLS Black/white[c]	2SLS Black[a]	2SLS White[b]	2SLS Black − white[c]	2SLS Black/white[c]
Black waterborne disease rate, 1911	144.2 (67.5)	Dep. var.				Dep. var.			
White waterborne disease rate, 1911	105.6 (38.9)		Dep. var.				Dep. var.		
Black − white	38.6 (53.7)			Dep. var.				Dep. var.	
Black/white	1.40 (0.51)				Dep. var.				Dep. var.
Miles of water mains per 100,000 persons[d]	132.3 (32.6)	−0.814* (2.20)	−0.409* (2.01)	−0.593* (2.02)	−0.004* (2.48)	−1.71* (1.75)	0.523 (0.420)	−0.641 (0.545)	−0.009 (0.782)
Black total death rate, except waterborne	2,533 (671)	0.051* (2.80)	...	0.043* (2.94)	0.001* (3.67)	0.047* (2.21)	...	0.043* (2.80)	0.001* (3.36)
White total death rate, except waterborne	1,540 (180)	...	0.097* (2.61)	−0.058 (0.93)	−0.001 (1.67)	...	0.192 (1.43)	−0.063 (1.08)	−0.001 (1.08)
Ave. waterborne disease rate, 1900	156.7 (63.7)	0.222 (1.28)	0.210* (3.16)	−0.174* (1.74)	−0.175* (1.98)	0.114 (0.51)	0.325* (1.83)	−0.180 (1.02)	−0.232 (1.37)
Constant	...	96.4 (1.19)	−27.4 (0.35)	128.6 (1.13)	2.50* (2.48)	238.3 (1.43)	−308.6 (0.807)	143.0 (0.398)	3.81 (1.11)
No. of observations	23	23	23	23	23	23	23	23	23
Adjusted R^2		0.409	0.657	0.354	0.386	0.226	0.276	0.352	0.288

Sources: See text.

Notes: t-Statistics are in parentheses. An asterisk indicates significant at the 10 percent level (two-tailed test).

[a] Regression weighted by black population.

[b] Regression weighted by white population.

[c] Regression weighted by total population.

[d] In two-stage regressions, fire hydrants per capita and ownership (i.e., whether public or private) of local gas and electric companies serve as instruments.

Table 8.3
Access to Water Service and Black and White Waterborne Disease Rates in 1915

Variable	Mean (S.D.)	OLS Black[a]	OLS White[b]	OLS Black − white[c]	OLS Black/white[c]	2SLS Black[a]	2SLS White[b]	2SLS Black − white[c]	2SLS Black/white[c]
Black waterborne disease rate, 1915	102.7 (58.1)	Dep. var.	...	...	...	Dep. var.	...	...	...
White waterborne disease rate, 1915	66.8 (29.6)	...	Dep. var.	...	...	...	Dep. var.	...	...
Black − white	35.8 (44.4)	...	...	Dep. var.	...	...	...	Dep. var.	...
Black/white	1.57 (0.744)	...	...	...	Dep. var.	...	...	...	Dep. var.
Percent of pop. connected to water[d]	91.2 (10.9)	−1.93* (2.15)	−0.057 (0.103)	−1.61* (2.14)	−0.023 (1.49)	−3.15* (2.08)	−0.622 (0.678)	−3.03* (2.26)	−0.037 (1.43)
Black total death rate, except waterborne	2,441 (470)	0.059* (3.76)	...	0.037* (2.49)	0.001 (1.40)	0.057* (3.52)	...	0.032* (1.95)	0.001 (1.16)
White total death rate, except waterborne	1,361 (167)	...	0.088* (3.35)	−0.032 (0.773)	−0.001 (0.514)	...	0.097* (3.35)	−0.008 (0.169)	−0.001 (0.119)
Ave. waterborne disease rate in 1900	1.49 (0.579)	0.307* (2.34)	0.243* (4.31)	0.179* (2.18)	0.226 (1.37)	0.349* (2.47)	0.246* (4.28)	0.190* (2.18)	0.238 (1.41)
Constant	...	94.0 (1.02)	−83.2 (0.19)	110.5 (1.46)	2.82* (1.85)	205.7 (1.42)	−41.6 (0.551)	221.8* (1.90)	3.96* (1.76)
No. of observations	35	35	35	35	35	35	35	35	35
Adjusted R^2		0.405	0.497	0.273	0.069	0.369	0.481	0.186	0.040

Sources: See text.
Notes: t-Statistics are in parentheses. An asterisk indicates significant at the 10 percent level (two-tailed test).
[a] Regression weighted by black population.
[b] Regression weighted by white population.
[c] Regression weighted by total population.
[d] In two-stage regressions, tons of garbage collected per capita and fire hydrants per capita serve as instruments.

Exploring the Effects of Segregation and Disease Spillovers

The 1908, 1911, and 1915 cross sections can also be used to explore the role of disease spillovers and residential segregation in shaping the relationship between waterborne disease rates and access to public water supplies. To explore the effects of segregation, the index of isolation was added to the regressions. (See chapters 3, 4, and 6 for discussions of the isolation index.) Presumably, if segregation reduced access to public services such as water and sewer lines, segregation would have been positively correlated with disease rates. There is some weak evidence in favor of this proposition. In the 1911 sample, black disease rates and the isolation index are positively and significantly correlated, although in all other samples the coefficient on the isolation index is small and statistically insignificant, perhaps in part because including the index requires dropping several observations for which data on segregation are not available. Nonetheless, it is important to note that in all of the samples, the inclusion of the isolation index does not alter the findings reported in tables 8.1, 8.2, and 8.3.

A more revealing approach for analyzing the effects of segregation involves dividing the full 1915 sample into two subsamples. As with the panel data in chapter 6, cities with an isolation index greater than or equal to the median value of this segregation index as of 1910 fall into one subsample and are called segregated cities, while cities with an index value less than the median fall into the other subsample and are called integrated cities.[2] The two subsamples can then be analyzed using the same procedures as those described here.

The results are reported in table 8.4. In segregated cities, variation in access to service clearly affected blacks disproportionately. The coefficient on percent connected is negative and significant for blacks and close to zero and insignificant for whites; moreover, variation in the percent connected reduced the difference between, and the ratio of, black and white disease rates. This suggests that in segregated cities, variation in mains mileage affected blacks disproportionately and that if water systems were incomplete, blacks alone (and not whites) were the ones to have gone without service. In contrast, in integrated cities, the ill effects of variation in service appear to have been distributed more equitably. The coefficient on percent connected is negative and significant for both blacks and whites; and variation in the percent connected had no effect on the difference between, or the ratio of, black and white disease rates. This suggests that in integrated cities, if water systems were incomplete, both blacks and whites went without service.[3]

Table 8.4
Segregation, Racial Disparities in Disease, and Connections to Public Water Systems in 1915

Variable	Segregated cities				Integrated cities			
	Black[a]	White[b]	Black – white[c]	Black/ white[c]	Black[a]	White[b]	Black – white[c]	Black/ white[c]
Percent of pop. connected to water[d]	−2.26* (2.30)	−0.268 (0.504)	−2.51* (3.65)	−0.041* (3.18)	−3.47* (1.78)	−1.89* (1.73)	−0.827 (0.438)	0.031 (0.613)
Black total death rate, except waterborne	0.049 (1.56)	...	0.023 (0.904)	0.001 (1.34)	0.054* (2.53)	...	0.063* (2.32)	0.001* (1.73)
White total death rate, except waterborne	...	0.107* (2.79)	0.029 (0.491)	−0.001 (0.252)	...	0.144* (2.61)	−0.080 (0.722)	−0.004 (1.17)
Waterborne disease rate in 1900	0.695* (3.66)	0.319* (3.71)	0.507* (3.86)	0.593* (2.44)	0.201 (1.20)	0.164* (1.74)	0.075 (0.487)	0.421 (1.01)
Constant	63.1 (0.505)	−110.7 (1.69)	82.4 (0.999)	3.04* (1.99)	261.7 (1.32)	5.81 (0.059)	61.0 (0.376)	0.071 (0.016)
No. of observations	14	14	14	14	13	13	13	13
Adjusted R^2	0.537	0.588	0.625	0.422	0.544	0.650	0.364	0.001

Sources: See text.

Notes: *t*-Statistics are in parentheses. An asterisk indicates significant at the 10 percent level (two-tailed test).

[a] Regression weighted by black population.

[b] Regression weighted by white population.

[c] Regression weighted by total population.

[d] In two-stage regressions, tons of garbage collected per capita and fire hydrants per capita serve as instruments.

Table 8.5 reports the results of a series of regressions looking at
spillovers. The first three identify the effect of black waterborne disease
rates on white rates. These regressions control for overall white mortality, the extensiveness of local water systems (miles of water mains
per 100,000 persons or percent connected to water system), and waterborne disease rates in 1900. They also assume that the black waterborne disease rate is endogenous; the total black mortality rate serves
as an instrument. In all three regressions, the coefficient on the black
waterborne disease rate is negative (the wrong sign) and insignificant.
This indicates that there were few spillovers in waterborne diseases
from black to white households, a finding that appears inconsistent
with the analysis of panel data in the previous section. One obvious
avenue of reconciliation focuses on the differences in the diseases
under consideration. The analysis of panel data employs only typhoid
rates while the analysis here employs all waterborne diseases, including various forms of diarrhea. It is possible that while there were spillovers for typhoid fever, no such spillovers existed for diarrhea.[4]

The final three regressions in table 8.5 support this proposition. In
the 1911 sample, the coefficient on black typhoid rates is positive and
significant at the 5 percent level in a one-tailed test; and in the 1915
sample, the coefficient is positive and significant at the 8 percent level
in a one-tailed test. These three regressions use total black mortality
rates (exlcuding waterborne diseases) as an instrument for black typhoid rates. Also, the results are unchanged if, rather than controlling
for the total waterborne disease rate in 1900, one controls only for the
typhoid rate observed in 1900.

8.3   Test Two

Estimation Strategy

The econometric work in this section builds on the following logic:
Suppose that cities responded to demand from white households and
neighborhoods for public water and sewer service, but did not respond to such a demand from black households and neighborhoods. If
this were the case, cities would have installed new water and sewer
mains in response to increases in the white population, but would have
refrained from installing new mains in response to increases in the
black population. If, however, cities were equally responsive to the
needs of black and white neighborhoods, new mains would have been
installed regardless of the race of newly added populations.

Table 8.5
Spillovers in the Cross-Sectional Data

Dependent variable	White waterborne disease rate[a]			White typhoid rate[a]		
Variable	1908 Sample	1911 Sample	1915 Sample	1908 Sample	1911 Sample	1915 Sample
Black waterborne disease rate[b]	−0.067 (0.518)	−0.567 (0.859)	−0.123 (0.415)	...	...	...
Black typhoid rate[b]	...	...	...	−0.615 (0.515)	0.684* (2.07)	0.590* (1.47)
White total death rate	0.126* (3.21)	0.192 (1.63)	0.110* (2.61)	0.020 (0.377)	0.012 (0.640)	−0.007 (0.453)
Waterborne disease rate in 1900	0.651* (5.75)	0.263* (1.96)	0.248* (1.95)	0.226 (1.15)	2.77 (0.804)	0.323 (1.16)
Miles of water mains per 100,000 persons	−12.1* (2.24)	−8.47 (1.25)	...	−6.06 (0.545)	−9.15 (0.731)	...
Percent of pop. connected to water system	...	...	−0.444 (0.520)	...	...	1.12 (0.210)
Constant	7.12 (0.069)	−45.2 (0.326)	−72.7 (1.20)	59.4 (0.264)	−9.37 (0.248)	4.05 (0.188)
No. of observations	15	23	35	15	23	35
Adjusted R^2	0.756	0.001	0.407	0.001	0.357	0.065

Sources: See text.
Notes: t-Statistics are in parentheses. An asterisk indicates significant at the 10 percent level (one-tailed test).
[a] Regression weighted by white population.
[b] The total black mortality rate excluding waterborne diseases serves as an instrument.

With this logic in mind, variants on the following regression equation are now estimated:

$$\Delta MAINS_i = \alpha + \beta_b \Delta BPOP_i + \beta_w \Delta WPOP_i + \delta_b BPOP0_i$$

$$+ \delta_w WPOP0_i + \gamma MAINS0_i + e_i, \qquad (8.4)$$

where $\Delta MAINS$ is the change in the miles of water mains installed in city i between t_0 and t_1; $\Delta BPOP$ ($\Delta WPOP$) is the change in city i's black (or white) population between t_0 and t_1; $BPOP0$ ($WPOP0$) is city i's black (or white) population at t_0; and $MAINS0$ is the miles of water mains city i had installed by t_0. The inclusion of miles of mains installed at t_0 controls for the initial size of the system. Presumably cities with already large water systems would have required fewer extensions than those with small systems.[5]

Equation (8.4) is estimated with two separate data sets. One covers the 1890–1900 period, the other the 1900–1920 period. The 1890–1900 sample consists of thirty-five southern towns and cities. The 1900–1920 sample consists of twenty-three large cities from across the United States. Table 8.6 gives descriptive statistics for these cities, which are listed in the table note. For the analysis that follows, it is important to note that the distribution of city size is skewed for both samples. For the white population in the 1890–1900 sample, the mean city in 1890 was nearly 5 times larger than the median city. For the white population in the 1900–1920 sample, the mean city in 1900 was 2.5 times larger than the median city. As for sources, data on mains mileage and growth in mains come from *The Manual of American Waterworks* and *The McGraw Directory of American Water Companies*. Data on population and population growth by race are from the associated decennial censuses of the U.S. Bureau of Census.

Once Eq. (8.4) has been estimated, the coefficients on $\Delta BPOP$ and $BPOP90$ can be compared with the coefficients on $\Delta WPOP$ and $WPOP90$ to see how growth in mains responded to variation in black and white populations. In particular, consider the following plausible hypotheses and the coefficient estimates they imply:

Hypothesis 8.5
Black neighborhoods received no water service before t_0, while white neighborhoods did. In this case, initial black population and black population growth would not have affected how many water mains cities installed. This implies the following coefficient estimates: $\beta_w \geq \beta_b = 0$; $\delta_w > \delta_b = 0$.

Table 8.6
Some Descriptive Statistics on Mains Mileage and Population

	1890–1900 Sample[a]			1900–1920 Sample[b]		
	Mean	Median	S.D.	Mean	Median	S.D.
$\Delta MAINS$	13.3	8.5	16.5	364	203	457
$\Delta BPOP$	502	369	4,945	22,783	13,980	25,885
$\Delta WPOP$	2,739	746	6,157	274,488	119,288	453,451
$BPOP0$	6,054	2,382	8,433	26,775	20,355	25,107
$WPOP0$	10,129	2,442	23,114	466,608	201,113	743,492
$MAINS0$	7.14	0	18.9	402	294	387
No. of observations	35	35	35	23	23	23

Sources: See text.
[a] The cities in the 1890–1900 sample are Albany, Ga.; Alexandria, La.; Americus, Ga.; Asheville, N.C.; Athens, Ga.; Atlanta, Ga.; Augusta, Ga.; Berkley, Va.; Brownsville, Tenn.; Clarksburgh, W.Va.; Covington, Ky.; Dalton, Ga.; Donaldsonville, La.; Fernandia, Fla.; Gainesville, Ga.; Grafton, W.Va.; Greenville, Miss.; Griffin, Ga.; Harrisonburg, Va.; Jackson, Tenn.; Key West, Fla.; Lebanon, Ky.; Lexington, Va.; Louisville, Ky.; Lynchburg, Va.; Manchester, Va.; Norfolk, Va.; Rome, Ga.; Savannah, Ga.; Thomasville, Ga.; Troy, Ala.; Valdosta, Ga.; Waycross, Ga.; Winston, N.C.; and Wytheville, Va.
[b] The cities in the 1900–1920 sample are New York, N.Y.; Chicago, Ill.; Philadelphia, Pa.; Detroit, Mich.; Cleveland, Ohio; St. Louis, Mo.; Boston, Mass.; Baltimore, Md.; Pittsburgh, Pa.; Buffalo, N.Y.; New Orleans, La.; Minneapolis, Minn.; Kansas City, Mo.; Providence, R.I.; Columbus, Ohio; Louisville, Ky.; Atlanta, Ga.; Toledo, Ohio; Richmond, Va.; Memphis, Tenn.; Dayton, Ohio; Hartford, Conn.; and Nashville, Tenn.

Hypothesis 8.6
Black neighborhoods received service after white neighborhoods, so that cities were responding to black population growth with a lag. In this case, while the growth of the white population would have prompted extensions in main mileage, growth in the black population would have prompted fewer extensions. Moreover, because cities responded with a lag to the needs of the black population, one expects initial black population levels to have influenced subsequent extensions in main mileage. This implies the following coefficient estimates: $\beta_w > \beta_b \geq 0; \delta_b > \delta_w \geq 0$.

Hypothesis 8.7
Black and white neighborhoods received service simultaneously; there was no discrimination. In this case, both black and white population growth would have prompted more extensions in main mileage and/or initial black and white population levels would have influenced

subsequent extensions in this mileage. This implies the following coefficient estimates: $\beta_b = \beta_w \geq 0$; and $\delta_b = \delta_w \geq 0$.

Hypothesis 8.8

A fourth hypothesis is suggested by the following caveat: Evidence presented in chapters 3, 4, and 5 indicates that blacks were often located on the periphery of cities and towns. Because these areas had relatively low population densities, providing peripherally located blacks with water service would have required more mains than providing service to centrally located whites. This biases the results in favor of finding no discrimination. Even in a world where blacks were getting less service than whites, the estimated coefficients on $\Delta BPOP$ and $BPOP90$ could appear similar to, or even larger than, the coefficients on $\Delta WPOP$ and $WPOP90$. In such a world, the coefficient estimates should be interpreted as establishing only a rough indicator of whether black neighborhoods had access to service. Coefficient estimates suggesting that public authorities were more responsive to variation in black population level and growth than they were to variation in white population level and growth (i.e., $\beta_b > \beta_w$ and $\delta_b > \delta_w$) would corroborate this view.

Results

Table 8.7 reports the regression results. Focusing on the regressions that include controls for population growth, the results contradict the hypothesis that black neighborhoods did not receive any water service during the 1890–1900 period or from 1900 to 1920. For the full 1890–1900 sample, increasing black population growth by a thousand persons generated an additional 0.6 mile of water mains; a similar increase for whites generated an additional 1.2 miles of mains. Increasing the initial black population by a thousand persons generated an additional 0.6 mile of water mains, while for whites it was 0.4 mile. While the point estimates themselves (ignoring standard errors) appear to be consistent with the hypothesis that cities responded to changes in the black population with a lag, one cannot reject the hypothesis that cities were equally responsive to the needs of both populations. More formally, one cannot reject the nulls, $\beta_b = \beta_w$ and $\delta_b = \delta_w$. This finding is consistent with the third hypothesis (8.7); there is no discrimination. For the full 1900–1920 sample, the results not only suggest that black neighborhoods received service, but that they received service faster

Table 8.7
How Growth in Water Mains Responded to Changes in Black and White Populations

	1890–1900 Sample					1900–1920 Sample			
	Full sample	Initial pop.	Pop. <60,000	Pop. <30,000	No mains	Full sample	Initial pop.	Pop. <1 million	Pop. <0.5 million
ΔMAINS	Dependent variable					Dependent variable			
ΔBPOP, β_b	0.0006* (4.03)	…	0.0007* (3.83)	0.0019* (2.04)	0.0017 (1.66)	0.0045* (2.30)	…	0.0023 (1.00)	0.0004 (0.17)
ΔWPOP, β_w	0.0012* (3.03)	…	0.0008 (1.47)	0.0002 (0.33)	0.0004 (0.13)	0.0003* (1.91)	…	0.0006* (2.86)	0.0006* (3.06)
BPOP0, δ_b	0.0006* (4.69)	0.0005* (3.73)	0.0006* (4.02)	0.0011* (2.36)	0.0012 (2.43)	0.0003 (0.26)	0.0008 (0.77)	0.0006 (0.76)	0.0021* (2.05)
WPOP0, δ_w	0.0004* (1.53)	0.0009* (5.04)	0.0004* (2.71)	0.0001 (0.61)	−0.0001 (0.29)	0.0004* (4.29)	0.0007* (14.8)	0.0010* (4.52)	0.0009* (3.99)
MAINS0	−0.342* (2.28)	−0.503* (2.10)	−0.336 (2.13)	−0.021 (0.09)	…	−0.366* (4.30)	−0.303* (3.60)	−0.885* (4.34)	−0.614* (3.03)
Constant	4.96* (7.16)	4.12* (3.61)	4.59* (5.92)	3.98* (4.17)	4.50* (4.16)	130.8* (3.93)	146.4* (3.54)	123.9* (4.34)	78.0* (2.23)
N	35	35	33	28	23	23	23	20	17
Adjusted R^2	0.967	0.904	0.768	0.474	0.430	0.969	0.940	0.744	0.762
Hypothesis tests	p-value					p-value			
$H_0 : \beta_b = \beta_w$	0.272	…	0.889	0.235	0.351	0.056	…	0.495	0.940
$H_0 : \delta_b = \delta_w$	0.420	0.070	0.421	0.180	0.081	0.899	0.918	0.677	0.308

Sources: See text.
Notes: t-Statistics are in parentheses. An asterisk indicates significant at the 10 percent level or higher (two-tailed test). Ellipses indicate not included in regression.

than white neighborhoods. Increasing black population growth by a thousand persons generated an additional 4.5 miles of water mains; a similar increase for whites generated only 0.3 mile. Increasing the initial black population by a thousand persons generated an additional 0.3 mile of water mains and for whites, 0.4 mile. The difference in the coefficient estimates on contemporaneous population change across races is statistically significant. This pattern is consistent with the fourth hypothesis (8.8).[6]

There are three concerns with these regressions. First, it is possible that population growth is endogenous. Although devising reasonable instruments in this case is fruitless, a remedial solution is available. In particular, white and black population growth can be dropped from the regressions and only initial population levels used. This procedure is identical to cross-country growth regressions that mitigate concerns about endogeneity by regressing growth rates against a series of initial conditions. For the 1890–1900 sample, dropping contemporaneous growth rates does not appear to alter the finding that blacks received service, although the coefficient on the initial black population is significantly smaller than that on the initial white population. For the 1900–1920 sample, the coefficients on black and white initial populations are qualitatively similar and statistically indistinguishable. (See the regressions labeled "Initial pop." in table 8.7 for results.)

Second, as noted earlier, the distribution of city size is highly skewed for both samples (see table 8.6). This raises the possibility that the effects of a few large cities swamp the effects of smaller cities. To test this possibility, regressions were also estimated over subsamples that excluded large cities. For the 1890–1900 sample, the two subsamples consisted of cities with total populations less than 60,000 or less than 30,000 persons in 1890. For the 1900–1920 sample, the two subsamples consisted of cities with total populations less than 1 million or a half million persons in 1900. For 1890–1900 data, the subsamples yield conclusions that are identical to the full 1890–1900 sample; one cannot reject the third hypothesis that cities responded similarly to the needs of blacks and whites. For the 1900–1920 sample, excluding large cities changes the results; for both subsamples, the results now support the third hypothesis of no discrimination (see table 8.7 for results).

Third, thus far it has been implicitly assumed that the technology of water distribution was such that adding one household to a water system required x miles of mains to have been installed, and that x was a constant positive number, regardless of the number of homes connected to the system. The assumption that x was constant over the number of households connected is a strong one and is probably unrealistic. A more realistic assumption is that x was a negative function of the number of households connected to the system, so that as the number of homes connected to the system rose, the miles of mains needed to connect a new home fell. Imagine then a world where cities had largely completed installing mains in all white neighborhoods, but were only just beginning to install mains in black neighborhoods. If one estimated Eq. (8.4) with data from such a world, the resulting coefficients on population level and growth would appear much larger for blacks than for whites, even though blacks were receiving service more slowly.

To address this concern, the 1890–1900 sample is restricted to towns that start the period with no water system, which represents well over half of the towns in the full sample. In the restricted sample, black and white neighborhoods would have clearly been at the same point in the development of their water systems; neither would have had any mains. If the sample is restricted to towns without any water mains in 1890, the results again support the third hypothesis (8.7) of no discrimination, so that one cannot reject the nulls, $\beta_b = \beta_w$ and $\delta_b = \delta_w$. Overall, it is notable that all but two of the nine regressions reported in table 8.7 are consistent with the hypothesis of no discrimination.

Exploring the Effects of Segregation and Disease Spillovers

By adding data on segregation and disease rates to Eq. (8.4), it is possible to explore how segregation and disease spillovers influenced access to public water systems. If segregation promoted unequal access, one expects that segregated cities would have exhibited less growth in water mains than integrated cities. The regression results for this approach are given in table 8.8. Using the 1900 index of isolation, there is strong evidence that cities with high levels of segregation exhibited significantly slower growth in mains (see regression 1, table 8.8). The negative correlation between segregation and growth in mains is robust to the inclusion of variables controlling for population density and southern location, and although the results are less strong, the same relationship appears to hold when the sample is restricted to southern cities (see regressions 2 and 3). One also expects that segregated cities would have been less responsive to black population increases, in terms of extending water mains, than integrated cities.

Table 8.8
Disease, Segregation, and Growth in Mains

	Regression						
	1	2	3	4	5	6	7
				Dependent variable			
ΔMAINS							
ΔBPOP	0.0056* (3.43)	0.0061* (3.49)	...	0.0104* (4.09)	0.0055* (3.40)	0.0058* (2.97)	0.0066* (4.01)
ΔWPOP	0.0003* (2.10)	0.0002* (1.74)	...	0.0002 (1.44)	0.0003* (1.99)	0.0019 (0.95)	0.0001 (1.04)
BPOP00	0.0006 (0.66)	−0.0004 (0.34)	0.0017 (0.82)	0.0002 (0.25)	0.0021 (1.24)	−0.0002 (0.19)	0.0001 (0.016)
WPOP00	0.0004* (4.92)	0.0004* (4.87)	0.0004 (1.80)	0.0003* (4.17)	0.0004* (4.87)	0.0004* (4.03)	0.0004* (5.92)
MAINS00	−0.366* (5.33)	−0.376* (5.07)	...	−0.290* (3.89)	−0.347* (4.90)	−0.388* (3.98)	−0.391* (5.94)
Density	...	0.0032 (0.71)	...	...	...	...	...
South	...	44.5 (0.86)	...	...	...	...	...
Segregation index	−14.2* (3.18)	−17.0* (3.21)	−10.7 (1.14)	−9.14 (1.08)	−6.34 (0.73)	...	0.510 (1.22)
Index × ΔBPOP	...	...	...	−0.030 (0.71)	...	...	...
Index × BPOP00	...	...	...	...	−0.027 (1.05)	...	7.78 (0.40)

Black disease	⋮	⋮	⋮	⋮	⋮	0.006 (0.04)	⋮
White disease	⋮	⋮	⋮	⋮	⋮	0.019 (0.04)	⋮
Index × black disease	⋮	⋮	⋮	⋮	⋮	⋮	−10.7 (1.25)
Constant	203.9* (5.76)	203.9* (5.76)	164.3 (1.14)	173.4* (3.09)	163.5* (3.13)	139.6* (1.95)	125.6 (1.21)
N	23	23	9	23	23	20	20
Adjusted R^2	0.980	0.980	0.411	0.979	0.980	0.965	0.985

Sources: See text.

Notes: t-Statistics are in parentheses. An asterisk indicates significant at the 10 percent level or higher (two-tailed test). Ellipses indicate not included in regression.

Regressions 4 and 5, however, yield at best weak evidence that more segregated cities were less responsive to changes in black population than integrated cities.

If fear of disease encouraged cities to extend water mains, growth in mains between 1900 and 1920 would have been positively correlated with disease rates in 1900; cities with high black and white waterborne disease rates would have invested in water mains more aggressively. The regression results in table 8.8 do not support this hypothesis. Neither black nor white disease rates in 1900 affected growth in mains over the subsequent 20 years (see regression 6). This finding is not altered by the following steps: restricting the sample of cities to those with populations less than 1 million or less than a half million; using total mortality rates instead of waterborne disease rates; using typhoid rates rather than waterborne disease rates; using dummy variables to capture unusually severe outbreaks of waterborne diseases; and using the proportion of all deaths attributable to waterborne diseases or typhoid instead of waterborne disease or typhoid rates. However, interacting segregation with black typhoid rates, there is very weak evidence that the fear of epidemic diseases spreading from black to white households was higher in integrated cities and prompted officials to extend service to blacks (see regression 7).

8.5   Conclusions

The econometric results from the first set of tests corroborate and expand on the findings in chapter 6. In particular, the results here show that in most cities black households were receiving water service, but only after white neighborhoods received this service. The evidence that blacks were receiving service with a lag is much stronger in segregated than in integrated cities; and in integrated cities, it appears that black and white households were receiving service concurrently. This finding constitutes one further piece of evidence that residential segregation facilitated efforts to deny blacks service, and conversely, that integration made it more likely that blacks received service roughly equal to that for whites. Finally, although they are not as strong as the evidence in chapter 6, the regression results provide some support for the idea that typhoid was transmitted across the color line.

The econometric procedures used in the second set of tests yield results that are more ambiguous than those reported in chapter 6. The findings here indicate that in terms of extending water lines, cities were as responsive to changes in the black population as they were to changes in the white population. This suggests there was minimal discrimination. The results for segregation and disease spillovers, however, are not particularly inspiring. There is some evidence that segregated cities exhibited slower growth in mains than integrated cities and perhaps were less responsive to changes in the black population. As for disease spillovers, or fear of disease, there is almost no evidence from these regressions that high disease rates prompted cities to extend water lines.

9   Conclusions

9.1 Summary of Findings

The central conclusion to emerge from this study is as follows: During the era of Jim Crow, there was less discrimination and inequality associated with the provision of public water and sewer facilities than one might otherwise expect, especially when one considers the widespread and severe discrimination that occurred in education, public parks, employment, police protection, and other public arenas. I have presented a mix of qualitative and quantitative evidence in support of this proposition. For qualitative evidence, in the case studies of Memphis, Tennessee, and Savannah, Georgia, I combine maps of local water and sewer systems with manuscript census data to recreate the geography of race and infrastructure in both cities around the turn of the twentieth century. In the case of Memphis, blacks were not substantially less likely than whites to have fronted streets with sewer mains around 1885. An analysis of mortality rates corroborates this finding. Black and white mortality rates in Memphis fell by about the same amount after the installation of sewers. In the case of Savannah, by 1905, 100 percent of all blacks and whites in the sample fronted streets with water mains. There is, however, some evidence of unequal access to sewers around 1900, and this inequality was related to residential segregation.

Other qualitative evidence includes the case studies of Pittsburgh, Pennsylvania, and Shaw, Mississippi. Pittsburgh is sometimes held up as the paradigmatic example of a highly segregated city that failed to install adequate water and sewer lines in poor immigrant and African-American neighborhoods. The analysis in chapter 3, however, shows that disease rates among blacks and foreign-born whites were no less responsive to the installation of a water filter in 1908 than rates among native-born whites. This finding suggests that there were no large racial disparities in access to the public water supply in Pittsburgh. The case study of Shaw builds on the idea that if discrimination in the provision of public water and sewer lines was as severe and widespread as it was in other areas, such as education and public parks, the amount of litigation regarding sanitation facilities would have been qualitatively similar to the amount of litigation surrounding schools and parks. The experience of Shaw and the two other municipalities (Arcadia and Fort Myers, Florida) that have been found guilty of providing unequal access to public water and sewer lines for existing black neighborhoods suggests that litigation of this variety is a rare event.

For quantitative evidence, I analyze seven independent data sources using four separate estimation strategies, and all of my findings point toward the same general conclusion. By the turn of the twentieth century, African-American households were not significantly less likely than white households to have had access to public water and sewer lines. Specifically, the analysis in chapters 6 and 7 demonstrates that when cities installed water filters, black typhoid rates were no less responsive to that improvement than were rates for whites. If blacks had had much less access to public water lines than whites, one would expect to see white typhoid rates falling while black rates remained constant. Chapter 8 explores how variation in the extensiveness of water systems affected black and white waterborne disease rates in cross sections of American cities in 1908, 1911, and 1915. The results suggest that black neighborhoods were receiving water lines a short time after white neighborhoods, but the results also show that black neighborhoods were indeed receiving service. One plausible explanation for the observed lag is that African Americans tended to locate in less densely populated peripheral areas and it took some time to extend mains from more densely populated areas located near the central part of cities.

The analyses in chapter 6 and to a lesser extent those in chapter 8, are predicated on the assumption that typhoid rates in a given city became increasingly responsive to improvements in the purity of water from the public system as an increasing proportion of the city's population was connected to public water lines. In chapter 7 I build a formal model to specify this assumption more precisely and then estimate the parameters of the model to see if this is in fact a justified assumption.

The empirical work suggests that the assumption is reasonable and that increasing access to public water lines also increased the responsiveness of waterborne disease rates to changes in water quality. I also implicitly test the validity of this key assumption by using measures of access other than disease rates to isolate inequities.

Rather than using disease rates as a proxy for access to service, some of the analysis in chapter 8 uses population levels and growth rates. This analysis is based on the idea that if cities were ignoring the needs of black neighborhoods, increases in the black population would not have induced cities to install additional water mains, while increases in the white population would have. The results do not support this hypothesis. Cities responded similarly in terms of installing new water mains to increases in the black and the white populations. Chapter 5 employs a large data set that consists of more than 250,000 households drawn from the Integrated Public Use Micro Data Series. Analysis of these data shows that in 1960, before the Civil Rights movement began and a decade before a federal court ruled against the town of Shaw, there were no large differences in the rates at which African-American and white households were connected to public water and sewer lines. In areas outside the South, there is even evidence that African-American households were somewhat more likely than white ones to have been connected to public water lines.

In at least one sense, the summary thus far understates the strength of my results. Specifically, the evidence in chapters 3 and 6 indicates that African-American households benefitted more than white households when cities installed water purification systems. Chapter 3 shows that the difference between black and (native-born) white typhoid rates in Pittsburgh fell from 140 deaths per 100,000 persons to less than 20 immediately after the city installed a water filter in 1908, and by 1920, racial disparities in typhoid rates had been almost entirely eliminated. In a more formal statistical analysis, chapter 6 shows that no matter how one measures racial disparities in typhoid rates, either differences or ratios, typhoid rates in the typical American city converged after a water filter was installed. More precisely, in the typical American city, installing a water filter reduced black typhoid rates by 53 percent, but reduced white rates by only 16 percent (see table 6.3). This finding is robust to most samples so that even in the South, improving water purification technologies reduced black typhoid rates by 44 percent while it reduced white rates by only 24 percent (see table

6.5). And as explained in chapter 7, the extent to which blacks benefitted disproportionately in the South is probably underestimated because of the tendency to conflate typhoid and malaria.

The evidence that blacks benefitted more than whites from water filtration prompts the question of why blacks gained more than whites. In chapter 3, building on the previous work of Koppes and Norris,[1] I argue that poor socioeconomic groups were disadvantaged in terms of their ability to prevent typhoid through private, household-level actions. As a result, white households, who were already preventing typhoid through private precautions, did not experience dramatic reductions in typhoid rates following public investments, while black households, who were not engaging in private prevention, depended heavily on public authorities to provide clean and safe water through public water lines.

I began this book with a puzzle: How was it that during the early twentieth century, a period of widespread discrimination against African Americans, black life expectancy improved so dramatically, both in absolute terms and relative to whites? One way to help resolve this puzzle is to recognize that there was limited discrimination in the provision of public water and sewer lines, and that blacks benefitted more than whites, in terms of disease reduction, from investments in water and sewer lines and water purification systems. Furthermore, as shown in chapter 2, providing clean water and proper sewage disposal not only eliminated typhoid and diarrhea, it promoted better overall health and helped reduce deaths from diseases that would not otherwise appear to have had a waterborne component.

The argument that there was limited discrimination in the provision of water and sewer lines inevitably prompts the question of why the inequalities associated with public water and sewer systems were so much less severe than in other public arenas, such as education. The key proposition here is that residential segregation was limited in turn-of-the-century America and this made it difficult to deny service to blacks without also denying service to whites. The low level of segregation also facilitated the spread of disease.

I present evidence on this issue in three chapters. In chapter 3, I cite the work of three prominent economists who have explored the evolution of residential segregation in American cities from 1890 through 1990.[2] Their work, as well as the work of others in allied disciplines, clearly shows that residential segregation was less pronounced in 1890 than it was 1970. The case studies of Memphis and Savannah in chapter 4, which adopt a fine geographic focus, support the idea that segregation was relatively limited in American cities around the turn of the century.

Evidence that residential integration undermined efforts to deny blacks water and sewer service is presented in several chapters. In chapter 4 I show that a city with a low level of residential segregation (Memphis) had a more extensive and racially equitable sewer system than a city with a relatively high level of segregation (Savannah). I show this by using maps of water and sewer systems and by comparing how disparities in black and white waterborne disease rates responded to improvements in these systems in both cities. In chapter 5 I use a few exceptional cases to make the point that segregation mattered. All of the municipalities in the United States that have been sued for refusing to provide black homeowners with adequate water and sewer services built their water and sewer systems late in the twentieth century, at a time when residential segregation was nearly complete.

Statistical evidence further buttresses the claim that integration undermined efforts to discriminate. The analysis of panel data in chapter 6 reveals that blacks gained much more from water filtration in integrated cities than in those that were segregated, suggesting that in segregated cities blacks had relatively limited access to public water lines. For example, the panel data showed that in integrated cities, water filtration reduced the waterborne disease rates for blacks by 57 percent, while in segregated cities it reduced these rates by less than half that amount (21 percent). Along the same lines, the analysis showed that in integrated cities, filtration reduced the ratio of black to white typhoid rates by 53 points, while in segregated cities, it *increased* the ratio by 3 points. The analysis in chapter 8 shows that variation in the extensiveness of water systems across cities had a much larger impact on disparities in disease rates in segregated than in integrated cities. This finding suggests that blacks were more likely to have been treated inequitably in segregated cities than in those that were integrated. Chapter 8 also provides some evidence that water systems were less extensive in segregated than in integrated cities.

Evidence on the significance of disease spillovers is presented in several chapters. It is useful to first review the statistical evidence on disease spillovers and then turn to the qualitative evidence. Accordingly, the analysis in chapter 6 provides strong and direct statistical evidence that typhoid was transmitted from black households to white ones. Indeed, nearly all of the benefits that whites realized from water filtration were indirect in the sense that filtration reduced the incidence of typhoid among black households, which in turn reduced the number of black-to-white transmissions of the disease. The findings in chapter 8, however, suggest that interracial disease spillovers occurred only in the case of typhoid and did not occur for other diarrheal diseases.

For qualitative evidence on disease spillovers, the experience of Memphis shows how fear of epidemic disease prompted some cities to install extensive and relatively equitable sewer systems. The experience of Jacksonville demonstrates how racism heightened white fears that diseases were spreading from black homes to their own, and drove public officials to advocate extending water and sewer lines to black neighborhoods.

Having said this, one might wonder if the statistical findings in chapter 6 support or validate, in any way, the repulsive views of doctors C. E. Terry and William Brunner. They do not. There is a clear difference between arguing that blacks had high disease rates because they were innately lazy and careless, as Terry and Brunner believed, and arguing that blacks had high disease rates because they were denied access to the same educational and employment opportunities as whites. Similarly, the statistical finding that diseases spread from poor and disadvantaged households to wealthy and advantaged ones reflects nothing more than the epidemiological tendency for diseases to spread from the ill, who were usually poor and members of a minority group, to the healthy, who were usually better off financially and white.

9.2   Connections

In a recent years historians have grown increasingly interested in the relationships among residential segregation, interracial disparities in disease and mortality rates, and the possibility that germs and disease were spread across the color line. There is particular interest in the accuracy of statements by public officials who claimed that diseases like cholera and typhoid originated in poor, foreign-born white, or African-American neighborhoods and spread to the relatively wealthy neighborhoods of native-born whites. There are also claims that the fear of epidemic disease prompted cities to segregate the races. For example, in his study of public health in Nashville, Tennessee, Don Doyle hypothesized that segregation was driven at least in part by fear of epidemic diseases spreading from black to white households.[3] In the responses to one of the papers delivered by Dr. C. E. Terry, one can find qualitative evidence to support this view.[4] The Achilles heel of this historical literature is not the absence of qualitative evidence, it is the absence of reliable statistical evidence on the magnitude of disease spillovers. By measuring the size of these spillovers, this study has provided a necessary first step in developing a more complete understanding of the role that disease played in shaping the urban landscape and in political decision making more generally.

Among economists, there are significant differences of opinion about the role of the state in a society. These differences stem not only from irreconcilable beliefs about what is right and wrong in a moral sense, but also from different empirical perceptions about the efficiency of markets. More precisely, for economists, there are two standard justifications for state intervention in a particular market: the presence of sizeable externalities or of increasing returns to scale (a natural monopoly), both of which generate market failures and make state intervention attractive. There are also differences of opinion about just how often market failures occur. For some persons, market failures are frequent and severe, and therefore a large and active government sector is desirable. For others, market failures are neither frequent nor severe, especially when compared with the only real-world alternative to market solutions: government intervention. Despite my sympathies for the latter view, the findings here bolster the case for government intervention at least in the case of supplying public water and sewer facilities. There were large and significant externalities associated with failing to provide these services, and when local governments intervened to provide them, health was improved for everyone. Typhoid was eliminated, and we no longer live in a world where we face a one-in-three chance of contracting that disease. The social returns on such interventions were enormous.[5]

Along the same lines, in *Competition and Coercion*, Robert Higgs argues that during the era of Jim Crow, market forces were the primary source of protection blacks had against racially unjust laws. Higgs also argues that the rapid improvements in black life expectancy that occurred during the late nineteenth and early twentieth centuries were primarily the result of improvements in the black standard of living. He expressly rejects the idea that public health improvements, such as improvements in water and sewer systems, played even a small role in improving African-American longevity.[6] In my view, the broader argument in Higgs—that market forces helped to minimize the adverse effects of racially unjust laws—has found ample support and documentation in subsequent research.[7] Higgs and I diverge only on his claim that public health interventions had little benefit for blacks. On this point, it is possible to restate my argument in a way that is at least consistent with the broader argument that Higgs offers. Markets, according to Higgs, minimized the adverse consequences of racist attitudes because they imposed costs on those individuals who chose to indulge their tastes for racism. In the case of public water and sewer systems, discrimination was minimized because it was costly to white politicians and voters. Disease spillovers, and the difficulty of denying blacks service in relatively integrated residential settings, made it costly for white politicians and voters to deny blacks water and sewer service.

Since the publication of McKeown's *The Modern Rise of Population*, there has been controversy about the role of public health interventions, such as the introduction of public water and sewer services, in promoting longer life and reduced mortality.[8] Recent research suggests that such interventions may have been even more important than McKeown originally claimed.[9] This book contributes to this debate in two ways. First, the calculations presented in chapter 3 imply that the installation of public water and sewer systems and the associated elimination of waterborne diseases account for at least 25 percent of the decline in total mortality observed in the United States between 1900 and 1940. Second, this book highlights the importance of looking beyond averages and at the effects of various public health interventions across socioeconomic groups. The results in chapter 6, for example, suggest that poor socioeconomic groups gained much more from the installation of public water and sewer systems than wealthier groups.

Appendix: The Negro Mortality Project

A.1 Introduction

In May 1896, a conference titled "Negro Mortality in Cities" was held at Atlanta University, one of the country's leading African-American universities. This conference gave rise to an ambitious project—referred to here as the Negro Mortality Project (NMP)—exploring why mortality among urban-dwelling blacks was so much higher than mortality among urban whites. The leaders of the project hoped that if the causes of excess black mortality were understood, effective public policies could be devised to bring black health in line with that of whites. Conducted jointly by Atlanta University and the U.S. Department of Labor, the NMP surveyed 1,137 African-American families, representing a total of 4,743 individuals during the year ending May 1897. The families lived mostly in the South, in cities and towns of all sizes; large cities such as Atlanta and Savannah in Georgia were covered, as were several small towns with populations less than 4,000.

The NMP culminated in an unusually detailed report that was published by the U.S. Department of Labor in 1897.[1] The final report included, among other things, household-level data on sickness during the past year; deaths and cause of death during the past 5 years; employment and earnings of father, mother, and children; occupation; schooling; cleanliness of household and surrounding neighborhood; and limited information about plumbing and access to running water and sewer lines. Despite the richness of this data source, to my knowledge there have been no previous attempts to analyze the NMP's findings, statistically or otherwise.

In this appendix I describe the methods and representativeness of the NMP surveys. After identifying some concerns, I then describe how these concerns are addressed and how they affect the findings reported in earlier chapters. The discussion focuses on two aspects of the NMP data. The first is the tendency of the NMP to survey clusters of households. The second aspect revolves around the tendency of doctors in 1897 to confuse typhoid fever and malaria.

A.2   Methods and Representativeness

Directed by prominent African Americans, the Negro Mortality Project was headed by George C. Bradford, a trustee of Atlanta University, and three other black men, all graduates of the university. These were Joseph E. Smith, a minister from Chattanooga, Tennessee; R. R. Wright, a college president in Savannah; and Butler R. Wilson, a lawyer from Boston, Massachusetts. To identify the causes of excess black mortality, the project launched a detailed, censuslike investigation of black households and neighborhoods in eighteen American cities. The process of surveying black households was conducted exclusively by African-American men on a voluntary basis. The interviewers were teachers, lawyers, ministers, and doctors, and all were graduates of one of three African-American universities: Atlanta University, Fisk University, or Berea College. Three hundred men were invited to act as census takers. Of these, a hundred accepted the invitation and volunteered to serve, but only fifty were able to complete their surveys in time to have their results included in the final report published by the U.S. Department of Labor.

Table A.1 lists the cities surveyed for the NMP. Except for Cambridge, Massachusetts, all of the cities were located in the South. A broad range of city sizes was included. The smallest towns—such as Macon, Mississippi; Orangeburg, South Carolina; Sanford, Florida; and Tuskegee, Alabama—had populations of less than 4,000 persons in 1890. The largest cities—Atlanta; Cambridge; Louisville, Kentucky; Nashville, Tennessee; and Washington, D.C.—had populations greater than 50,000. When investigators canvassed these cities and towns, they did not attempt to survey all African-American households. Rather, they selected narrowly defined clusters "of ten to twenty houses standing together in the portions of the city which were thought to be representative of the various conditions of the Negro in that locality."[2] For example, in Atlantla, sixteen clusters were surveyed. One cluster was located on Auburn Avenue in the fourth ward, while another was located on Green's Ferry Avenue and Chapel Street on the city's west

Table A.1
Summary of the Negro Mortality Project

| City | Number surveyed | | | City population, 1890 | | Public water and sewers: % connected | | | |
| | Clusters | Families | People | Population | % Surveyed | NMP estimate 1897 | Census estimates[a] | | |
							1890	Midpoint	1909
Athens, Ga.	1	16	73	8,637	0.0084	0.063	n.a.	n.a.	n.a.
Atlanta, Ga.	16	324	1,292	65,514	0.0197	0.128	0.253	0.421	0.589
Birmingham, Ala.	2	17	63	26,178	0.0024	0.000	0.452	0.554	0.656
Cambridge, Mass.	1	98	360	70,082	0.0051	0.979	n.a.	n.a.	0.937
Cartersville, Ga.	1	10	53	3,171	0.0167	0.000	n.a.	n.a.	n.a.
Chattanooga, Tenn.	1	21	89	29,100	0.0020	0.000	n.a.	n.a.	0.871
Columbia, S.C.	3	15	81	15,353	0.0053	0.000	n.a.	n.a.	n.a.
Jackson, Tenn.	1	22	67	10,039	0.0067	0.000	0.309	n.a.	n.a.
Jacksonville, Fla.	3	77	327	17,201	0.0073	0.359	0.226	0.486	0.746
Louisville, Ky.	1	15	70	161,129	0.0004	0.000	0.400	0.656	0.912
Macon, Ga.	4	30	90	22,746	0.0040	0.000	n.a.	n.a.	0.845
Macon, Miss.	1	17	64	1,565	0.0409	0.235	n.a.	n.a.	n.a.
Nashville, Tenn.	10	246	1,090	76,168	0.0143	0.004	n.a.	n.a.	0.639
Orangeburg, S.C.	2	22	109	2,964	0.0367	0.000	n.a.	n.a.	n.a.
Sanford, Fla.	1	24	116	2,016	0.0575	0.125	n.a.	n.a.	n.a.
Savannah, Ga.	5	96	380	43,174	0.0088	0.012	0.499	0.559	0.618
Tuskegee, Ala.	2	21	119	1,803	0.0660	0.157	n.a.	n.a.	n.a.
Washington, D.C.	4	66	293	230,392	0.0013	1.000	0.984	0.952	0.919

Sources: U.S. Department of Labor, "Condition of the Negro" and Baker, *Waterworks*.
Notes: [a] n.a., data not available. Census estimates are for entire population, not only African Americans.

side. In Chattanooga, Tennessee, only one cluster was surveyed and it was located on East Eighth Street in the seventh ward.

This process of surveying homes clustered in tiny geographic areas raises concerns about the representativeness of the samples. Consider, for example, the sample of African-American homes drawn from Savannah. The investigators focused on four predominately black neighborhoods, including Yamacraw, and Southville. In terms of the map of Savannah presented in chapter 4 (figure 4.3), the four areas surveyed correspond to the exclusively black neighborhoods labeled 1, 2, 3, and 4. No African-American households located in more integrated areas of the city were surveyed. As shown in chapter 4, access to sewers was highly correlated with residential integration. In areas of the city where blacks and whites lived in close proximity to one another, blacks had sewers; in areas were blacks were isolated, they did not. Because investigators surveyed only clusters of homes in segregated areas, their results understate black access to public sewer lines in Savannah.

In their final report, the organizers of the NMP recognized the potential biases associated with surveying small clusters of homes and offered the following discussion and caveats: The authors believed that the surveys of Atlanta, Cambridge, and Nashville covered broad and diverse geographic areas and therefore generated reliable and representative portrayals of African-American life in these cities. They wrote:

Great care was taken in the selection of groups [clusters] and in securing data in Atlanta, Ga., Nashville, Tenn., and in Cambridge, Mass., and it is to the tabulation of these cities that we must look for the most representative and accurate showing of the condition of the negro so far as this investigation is concerned.[3]

The same could not be said for the other cities surveyed: "The data for the ... other cities have doubtless been gathered with ... as much care in most cases, but the same care could not be exercised in the *selection* of the 32 groups [in these cities] as [was the case] in [Atlanta, Cambridge, and Nashville]."[4]

There are at least three ways to address the concern about representativeness. First, we might focus exclusively on the results for Atlanta, Cambridge, and Nashville, the three cities the organizers were confident provided an accurate and representative sample of African-American life. Second, we can assess the nature and magnitude of bias by comparing the data from the NMP with that from more comprehensive and objective sources, such as the U.S. Census. For example, one might ask whether low-wage occupations are overrepresented in the NMP relative to census data. Third, we might focus on questions in which the social and demographic characteristics of the sample are a secondary concern. For example, in estimating the effects of access to public water and sewer lines on black morbidity, the representativeness of the sample's wage distribution would not be a substantial concern as long as we adequately control for wage differences across families.

A.3   Connections to Public Water and Sewer Lines

Table A.1 gives the proportion of African-American homes connected to public water and sewer lines according to the surveys conducted by the Negro Mortality Project. The results for each city are reported in the column labeled "NMP estimate, 1897." Connections to public water and sewer lines varied greatly across municipalities. In eight cities— Birmingham, Alabama; Cartersville, Georgia; Chattanooga, Tennessee; Columbia, South Carolina; Jackson, Tennessee; Louisville; Macon, Georgia; and Orangeburg—none of the African-American households surveyed were connected to public water and sewer lines. In five cities—Atlanta; Jacksonville, Florida; Macon, Mississippi; Sanford; and Tuskegee—between 10 and 40 percent of the African-American households surveyed had public water and sewer connections. In two cities—Cambridge and Washington—more than 95 percent of households surveyed had public water and sewer connections.[5]

As explained earlier, there is a concern about the representativeness of the samples drawn for the NMP and it is not clear, a priori, whether the estimates reported in table A.1 understate or overstate access to public water and sewer lines among African-American families. Figure A.1 helps us assess the direction and magnitude of the bias by relating the NMP survey estimates to an objective and comprehensive measure of the size of municipal water systems. Specifically, figure A.1 plots the estimated proportion of (African-American) households connected to public water and sewer lines in each city against the number of water taps per capita in each city. Data on the number of water taps in each city are from the 1897 volume of *The Manual of American Waterworks*, and city-level data on (total) population are from the 1890 census. (There are some cities for which data on water taps are not available and these are excluded from the analysis.) If the NMP surveys

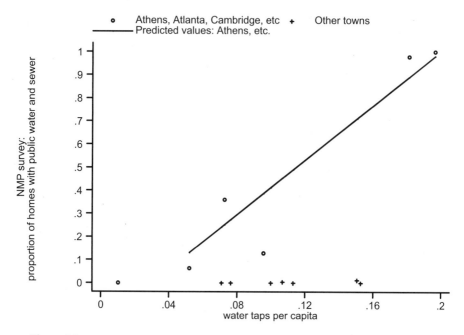

Figure A.1
Water taps per capita and connections to public water and sewer lines. Sources: U.S.
Department of Labor, "Condition of the Negro" and Baker, *Waterworks*.

accurately reflected the extensiveness of public water lines in African-
American neighborhoods, we would expect the proportion of households connected to rise as the number of water taps per capita rose
because an increasing number of water taps per capita implies increasing connections to public water and sewer lines.

For a few cities, the relationship between proportion connected and
water taps per capita appears reasonable. This is particularly true of
Washington and Cambridge. In both cities there was one water tap for
every five persons, and in both cities 95 percent of African-American
households surveyed were connected to public water and sewer lines.
Considering that in 1900 the typical family had four to five members,
and that many families lived in dwellings with shared baths, one water
tap for every five persons implies near-universal connection to public
water lines.[6] This logic is borne out by data from the 1915 volume of
the U.S. Bureau of the Census's *General Statistics of Cities*, a more comprehensive source than the NMP surveys. These data are plotted in
figure A.2. According to the *General Statistics of Cities*, once there was

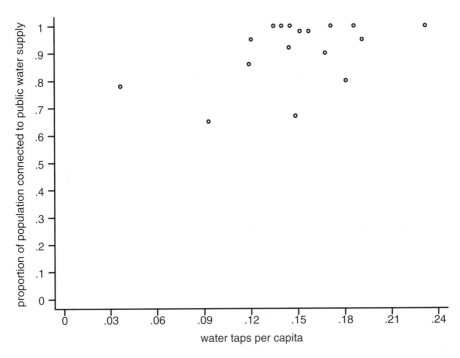

Figure A.2
Water taps per capita and connections to public water. Source: U.S. Bureau of Census, *General Statistics of Cities*, 1915. Data prepared by Center for Population Economics, University of Chicago.

one water tap for every four or five persons (in the general population), there was near-universal connection to public water supplies. Even in cities in which there was one water tap for every eight or nine persons, 80 percent or more of the total local population was typically connected to public water lines.

Returning to figure A.1, if one focuses exclusively on six cities—Orangeburg; Athens, Georgia; Jacksonville; Atlanta; Cambridge; and Washington—the relationship between estimated connection rates and water taps per capita is clearly linear and positive. In the remaining cities, no such correlation appears, and an increase in the number of water taps per capita has no effect on the estimated proportion of African-American households connected to public water and sewer lines. For these cities, the NMP surveys appear to understate connections to public water and sewer lines. For example, in Savannah in 1897, there was one water tap for every seven persons and by 1905 nearly the entire population of the city fronted streets with public water lines (see chapter 4), yet the NMP survey suggests that less than 2 percent of African-American households had access to public water and sewer lines. Excluding cities like Savannah would yield a more accurate portrayal of African-American access to water and sewer lines around 1900.

Some simple quantile regressions help formalize and sharpen this argument. More precisely, I regress the NMP estimates of connections to water and sewer lines in particular cities against water taps per capita in those same cities. I run separate regressions for the 90th, 80th, 70th, 60th, and 50th (median) percentiles, and then calculate the predicted values for each city. The argument developed in the preceding paragraphs suggests that the estimated relationship between water taps and connections to public water would have been most accurate for cities on the upper end of the distribution (e.g., the 80th and 90th percentiles) and less accurate for cities toward the middle and bottom end of the distribution. Quantile regressions for the 90th and 80th percentiles give greater weight to the city-level observations based on more accurate surveys and less weight to those based on less accurate surveys.

Table A.2 contains the regression results and the associated predicted values for each city. Notice first that the explanatory power is much higher for the 90th and 80th percentiles than it is for the 50th (median) percentile. This confirms the pattern observed in figure A.1— that only in cities on the upper end was variation in water taps per capita reflected in increased connections to public water. Notice also that the predicted values for the 90th and 80th percentiles are (not surprisingly) much larger than those for the 50th percentile. Consider, for example, the experience of Macon, the city with the median predicted value for all quantile regressions. Rather than having no African-American households connected to public water and sewer lines, as the NMP survey suggested, the regressions for the 80th percentile suggest that about 40 percent of all African-American households in the city were connected to public water and sewer lines in 1897. Are the predictions wrought by these upper-level percentiles reasonable? The results for Savannah suggest that they are. Recall that in chapter 4 it was shown that about 60 percent of all African-American homes in the city fronted streets with sewer mains. The predicted values for Savannah using the 70th and 80th percentiles are not far from this mark.

Table A.2
Water Taps per Capita and Access to Public Water and Sewer Lines

	Quantile regressions				
City-level variables	0.9	0.8	0.7	0.6	0.5
		Dependent variable			
Percent of black homes with public water and sewer connections					
Number of water taps per person	5.72* (0.392)	5.38* (2.48)	6.50* (2.93)	1.50 (5.50)	0.085 (2.02)
Pseudo R^2	0.556	0.457	0.234	0.049	0.006
Number of observations	13	13	13	13	13

City	Water taps per capita	NMP estimate	Predicted access from quantile regressions				
			0.9	0.8	0.7	0.6	0.5
Orangeburg, S.C.	0.010	0.000	0.000	0.000	0.000	0.000	0.000
Athens, Ga.	0.052	0.063	0.242	0.224	0.063	0.062	0.004
Cartersville, Ga.	0.071	0.000	0.350	0.326	0.185	0.091	0.005
Jacksonville, Fla.	0.073	0.359	0.359	0.335	0.196	0.093	0.005
Jackson, Tenn.	0.076	0.000	0.381	0.355	0.220	0.099	0.006
Atlanta, Ga.	0.096	0.128	0.491	0.460	0.346	0.128	0.007
Macon, Ga.	0.100	0.000	0.515	0.482	0.373	0.134	0.007
Nashville, Tenn.	0.107	0.004	0.555	0.519	0.419	0.144	0.008
Louisville, Ky.	0.113	0.000	0.591	0.552	0.459	0.154	0.009
Savannah, Ga.	0.151	0.012	0.805	0.754	0.703	0.210	0.012
Birmingham, Ala.	0.153	0.000	0.818	0.766	0.717	0.213	0.012
Cambridge, Mass.	0.181	0.979	0.979	0.917	0.900	0.255	0.014
Washington, D.C.	0.196	1.000	1.000	1.000	1.000	0.278	0.016

Source: See text.
Notes: Standard errors are in parentheses. An asterisk indicates significant at the 10 percent level or higher (one-tailed test).

Table A.3
Incidence of Waterborne Disease among NMP Households

City	Proportion of population ill from						
	Diarrhea	Dysentery	Typhoid	Malaria	Fever[a]	Total	Total − Malaria
Athens, Ga.	0.000	0.014	0.014	0.151	0.000	0.178	0.027
Atlanta, Ga.	0.002	0.002	0.007	0.040	0.012	0.062	0.022
Birmingham, Ala.	0.016	0.016	0.000	0.000	0.000	0.032	0.032
Cambridge, Mass.	0.008	0.000	0.014	0.003	0.008	0.033	0.030
Cartersville, Ga.	0.019	0.000	0.000	0.000	0.057	0.075	0.075
Chattanooga, Tenn.	0.000	0.000	0.000	0.022	0.011	0.034	0.011
Columbia, S.C.	0.000	0.000	0.000	0.222	0.000	0.222	0.000
Jackson, Tenn.	0.000	0.000	0.000	0.119	0.015	0.134	0.015
Jacksonville, Fla.	0.000	0.003	0.000	0.049	0.000	0.052	0.003
Louisville, Ky.	0.000	0.014	0.000	0.014	0.000	0.029	0.014
Macon, Ga.	0.000	0.011	0.000	0.156	0.011	0.178	0.022
Macon, Miss.	0.000	0.016	0.000	0.140	0.000	0.156	0.016
Nashville, Tenn.	0.006	0.001	0.005	0.047	0.009	0.067	0.020
Orangeburg, S.C.	0.000	0.000	0.000	0.110	0.000	0.110	0.000
Sanford, Fla.	0.000	0.000	0.000	0.371	0.000	0.371	0.000
Savannah, Ga.	0.000	0.000	0.000	0.139	0.003	0.142	0.003
Tuskegee, Ala.	0.000	0.000	0.000	0.067	0.000	0.067	0.000
Washington, D.C.	0.000	0.000	0.000	0.017	0.000	0.017	0.000
Average	0.003	0.004	0.002	0.093	0.007	0.109	0.016
Weighted average	0.003	0.002	0.004	0.064	0.007	0.080	0.016

Source: U.S. Department of Labor, "Condition of the Negro."
Notes: [a] fever of unknown cause.

A.4   Incidence of Waterborne Disease among African-American Families

Table A.3 reports the incidence of waterborne diseases among African-American populations surveyed by the NMP. A person is counted as ill from diarrhea, dysentery, fever of unknown cause, typhoid, and malaria if she or he told the NMP investigator that she or he had been sick with any of these illnesses during the previous year. Before describing the data, one needs to stress that these disease rates are imprecise. Individuals were self-reporting and based their answer on either a diagnosis from a doctor or their own best guess as to what had afflicted them during the past year. Since African Americans had limited access to high-quality medical care, one expects that there was a high degree of error associated with these diagnoses.

In the typical city, counting malaria as a waterborne disease increases the incidence rate by a factor of seven. As explained in chapter 7, typhoid was often mistakenly diagnosed as malaria, and it is reasonable to assume that nearly all cases of malaria were in fact typhoid. Because illnesses were self-reported and often self-diagnosed, the potential risk that typhoid was mistakenly referred to as malaria seems particularly large for the NMP data.

Notes

Chapter 1

1. For Gavin Wright's views on the Civil Rights movement, see Wright, "Revolution." On changes in black and white wage differentials and employment opportunities, see Donohue and Heckman, "Episodic Change." For data on home ownership, crime rates, and school attendance, see Collins and Margo, "Home Ownership"; the data appendices in Murray, *Losing Ground*, pp. 241–63; and U.S. Bureau of Census, *Historical Statistics*, p. 380. For data on improvements in poverty during the 1960s and onward, see Slesnick, "Gaining Ground."

2. Trends in white life expectancy are similar, although the change in trend around 1960 is much less pronounced. White life expectancy increased by about 30 percent between 1900 and 1940, and much less so during the 40-year period between 1960 and 2000. Also, demographers will notice immediately that much of the improvement in life expectancy, for both blacks and whites, stemmed from reductions in infant mortality. The primary killer of infants was diarrhea, a waterborne disease. This issue, and the sources of improvements in life expectancy more generally, are discussed in detail in chapters 2 and 4. See also Armstrong et al. "Trends"; Preston and Haines, *Fatal Years*; Elo and Preston, "African-American Mortality"; Ewbank, "Black Mortality"; and the following articles by Haines: "Ethnic Differences," "Estimated Life Tables," and "Urban Mortality Transition."

3. In the average city, black mortality rates fell by 8.8 deaths per 1,000 persons (30 percent), while white mortality rates fell by 6 deaths per 1,000 (32 percent). An important question here is how to best measure changes in relative mortality. That is, does one look at changes in percentages (the ratio of black to white death rates), or does one look at changes in levels (the difference between black and white death rates)? Clearly, the results in table 1.2 suggest the choice of metric can matter. This issue is examined in detail in chapter 7. The analysis there suggests that for the concerns addressed in this book, the absolute change (changes in differences), as opposed to the percentage change (changes in ratios), is the appropriate metric.

4. For information on lynching, see Tolnay and Beck, *Violence* and Brundage, *Lynching*. For the debate regarding income and wealth acquisition among blacks at the turn of the century, see Higgs, "Accumulation" and Margo, "Comment." It is true, however, that the late nineteenth and early twentieth centuries witnessed tremendous improvements in literacy rates among African Americans, both in absolute terms and relative to whites. See Margo, *Schooling*, pp. 5–8 and U.S. Bureau of Census, *Historical Statistics*, p. 382. Margo argues that the improvement in black literacy represents "pure catch up," with

African-American parents more likely to send their children to school than white parents, even after controlling for income and school quality.

5. Tomes, *Gospel of Germs*, p. 185.

6. Russell, *Atlanta*, pp. 156–60 and a related article, "Municipal Services."

7. See Hoffman, "Progressive Public Health."

8. See, for example, Doyle, *New Men*, pp. 281–84; Galishoff, "Germs"; Lineberry, *Municipal Services*; and Rabinowitz, *Race Relations*, pp. 121–23. To date, probably the most optimistic statement regarding access to public health facilities among poor socioeconomic groups is a doctoral dissertation by Gerard Fergerson, "Poor but Healthy."

9. All quotations are from Higgs, *Competition*, pp. 22–23.

10. Linder and Grove, *Vital Statistics*, pp. 330–35; and Troesken, "Race and Disease."

11. See, for example, Tomes, *Gospel of Germs*, p. 186; Ellis, *Yellow Fever*, pp. 113–15; Wrenn, "Sewer Experiment"; Russell, *Atlanta* and "Municipal Services"; Galishoff, "Germs"; Doyle, *New Men*, pp. 281–84; Rabinowitz, *Race Relations*, pp. 121–23; and Beardsley, *Neglect*. For statistical and demographic approaches to this general issue, see Ewbank, "Black Mortality," who argues that persistent differences in black mortality from typhoid and tuberculosis during the early twentieth century were probably driven by discrimination in the provision of health care. See also Preston and Haines, *Fatal Years*, who show that even after controlling for income, occupation, literacy, and the like, there were still large and unexplained differences in infant mortality rates between blacks and whites in 1900. Demographers and economists often attribute such unexplained differences to discrimination.

12. See U.S. Bureau of Census, *Historical Statistics*, p. 12. The data cited in this paragraph are merely suggestive. The definitions of urban areas have changed over time and the data in the text have not been adjusted to reflect this fact.

13. Quoted in Gadgil, "Drinking Water," p. 4.

14. See Szreter, "Social Intervention" and "Economic Growth." In "Economic Growth," Szreter presents evidence that unfettered economic development adversely affects health by promoting crowding in urban areas and thereby creating large problems in terms of sewage disposal and impure water, and other sorts of externalities that undermine health.

15. For another interpretation of the efficacy of public health interventions, see Condran and Crimmins-Gardner, "Public Health Measures."

16. For examples, see Rabinowitz, *Race Relations*, pp. 120–21; Galishoff, "Germs"; and Markel, "Cholera."

Chapter 2

1. Cholera was a rare event in the United States by 1900. For evidence on this, see any of the volumes of U.S. Bureau of Census, *Mortality Statistics*, between 1900 and 1920. There were, however, famous cholera epidemics in New York during the 1890s, and the broader United States during the mid-nineteenth century. See Markel, "Cholera"; Rosenberg, *Cholera*; and Fogel, *Without Consent*, pp. 360–65.

2. As noted in the introduction, previous studies developing this argument include McKeown, *Modern Population* and Szreter, "Social Intervention."

3. See Blake, *Water*; Budd, "Typhoid Fever"; Kiple, *Disease*, pp. 1071–76; Koppes and Norris, "Ethnicity"; Levy and Tuck, "Maggot Trap"; Tarr, *Ultimate Sink*, pp. 112–16; Clarence E. Smith, "Sanitary Privy"; Terry, "House Fly"; and Whipple, *Typhoid*, pp. 1–6.

4. See Curschmann, *Typhoid Fever*, pp. 33–72 and Whipple, *Typhoid*, pp. 1–6.

5. At one point, public health authorities in New York had Mallon committed. Despite an appeal to the U.S. Supreme Court, Mallon was not released until she promised to quit working as a cook. Shortly after her release, though, officials discovered her working as a cook in New Jersey. This time Mallon was locked away in a public institution for the rest of her life. See *New York Times*, November 12, 1938, p. 17 and Leavitt, *Typhoid Mary*.

6. Kiple, *Disease*, pp. 1071–76.

7. See Cain and Rotella, "Death and Spending"; Kiple, *Disease*, pp. 1071–76; Pritchett and Tunali, "Stranger's Disease"; and Whipple, *Typhoid*, pp. 1–6.

8. Curschmann, *Typhoid Fever*, pp. 37–42; Kiple, *Disease*, pp. 1071–74; Sedgwick, *Sanitary Science*, pp. 166–68; and Whipple, *Typhoid*, pp. 1–6. On the incidence of abdominal rashes, see Stephens and Levine, "Typhoid in Children."

9. Curschmann, *Typhoid Fever*, pp. 37–42; Kiple, *Disease*, pp. 1071–74; Sedgwick, *Sanitary Science*, pp. 166–68; and Whipple, *Typhoid*, pp. 1–6. On the neuropsychiatric effects of typhoid in modern-day populations, see Ali et al., "Neuropsychiatric Complications."

10. Khosla, "The Heart." See also, Buck and Simpson, "Infant Diarrhoea."

11. Costa, "Understanding Decline." In a more recent paper, however, Costa finds that exposure to typhoid during the Civil War did not affect overall mortality rates for mid- and older-age veterans. See Costa, "Understanding Mid-Life Mortality."

12. Whipple, *Typhoid*, p. 6.

13. Whipple, *Typhoid*, p. 3.

14. Costa, "Understanding Decline."

15. Costa, "Understanding Decline."

16. See Lindholt et al., "Review" for a survey of the evidence.

17. See Khosla, "Typhoid Hepatitis" and Morgenstern and Hayes, "The Liver." See also Kant Panday et al., "Typhoid and Hepatitis E," and Le et al., "Typhoid and Hepatitis."

18. See Khosla and Lochan, "Renal Dysfunction" and Adu et al., "Acute Renal Failure."

19. See Mathai et al., "*Salmonella typhi*."

20. See Ali et al., "Neuropsychiatric Complications."

21. See Budd, "Typhoid Fever"; Szreter, "Economic Growth"; Kiple, *Disease*, pp. 1073–75; and Melosi, *Sanitary City*, pp. 1–43, 60–61, and 110–13.

22. See Kiple, *Disease*, pp. 1077–80; Dale C. Smith, "Typhomalarial Fever"; and Whipple, *Typhoid*, pp. 1–6.

23. See U.S. Bureau of Census, *Mortality Statistics*, for the state of Mississippi.

24. For a racist statement on the inferiority of black doctors and health-care workers, see Terry, "The Negro," especially pp. 303–04. Similar statements can be found in the

discussions of typhoid fever in U.S. Bureau of Census, *Mortality Statistics*. For a scientific essay exploring the tendency to conflate typhoid and malaria, see Smith, "Typhomalarial Fever."

25. According to Whipple, *Typhoid*, p. 5, "good nursing, proper diet and hygiene, and the free use of the cold bath, [affected] a cure in from 90 to 95 percent of all cases." See also Kiple, *Disease*, pp. 1071–76.

26. Townsend, "Anti-Typhoid," p. 998.

27. The military's vaccination campaign was prompted by its experience during the Spanish-American War, when one in five American soldiers contracted typhoid fever. Six times as many soldiers died of typhoid than from war wounds. See American Water Works Association, *Manual*, pp. 15–25; Kiple, *Disease*, pp. 1071–76; and Whipple, *Typhoid*, pp. 1–6.

28. North Carolina State Board of Health, *Biennial Report*, 1889, p. 166.

29. North Carolina State Board of Health, *Biennial Report*, 1898, p. 47.

30. Mills, "Typhoid Fever," p. 151.

31. See U.S. Bureau of Census, *General Statistics of Cities*, 1907, pp. 131–372. The data given here exclude New York City.

32. See Troesken, "Race"; Baker, *Waterworks*, pp. 273–75; U.S. Bureau of Census, *General Statistics of Cities*, various years; and Elms, "Disinfection."

33. For other examples and evidence on the benefits of filtration, see Galishoff, *Newark*, pp. 185–87 and Tarr, *Ultimate Sink*, p. 236. For a more general statistical analysis of the benefits of installing water filters, see Cain and Rotella, "Death and Spending." Cain and Rotella also provide a detailed survey of the historical literature on urban infrastructure and typhoid rates. Meeker in "Social Return" finds that the social rate of return on investments in sewer and water filtration systems was enormous, perhaps as high as 150 percent. Another way to appreciate the benefits of water filtration is to note the strikingly large amount that wastewater filtration and purification plants treated. Consider, for example, this excerpt from a 1914 report by the water and sewerage board of New Orleans: "During the year 8,147 million gallons [of water] were treated at the Corolton plant, and 295 million gallons at the Algiers plant. This amount of water carried 21,300 tons of suspended matter, all of which was removed, and 3,800 tons of hardening constituents, about one-half of which was removed. Three thousand and fifty-eight tons of lime and 188 tons of sulphate of iron were required to soften and prepare the water for filtration." Quoted in U.S. Bureau of Census, *General Statistics of Cities* for the year 1915, p. 44. See also Sedgwick, *Sanitary Science*, pp. 187–94, 211–14, and 298–303; and Higgs, "Cycles and Trends."

34. See generally the following studies of infant mortality conducted by the U.S. Department of Labor, Children's Bureau: *Field Study in Manchester, Children of Preschool Age in Gary*, and *Results of a Field Study in Baltimore*. These studies were conducted between 1915 and 1923.

35. See U.S. Department of Labor, Children's Bureau, *Results of a Field Study in Baltimore*.

36. During the mid-1890s, the diarrheal death rate fell sharply, from approximately 220 deaths per 100,000 to just over 150. This unexplained drop occurred simultaneously with a drop in typhoid rates, suggesting that typhoid and diarrhea had a common environ-

mental source, which in this case was probably impure water. Indeed, using ward-level data from seventeen American cities in 1890, Higgs and Booth in "Mortality Differentials" find that typhoid fever rates and infant death rates were highly and significantly correlated. For typhoid rates in Pittsburgh over the late nineteenth and early twentieth centuries, see chapter 3 in general and figure 3.3 in particular.

37. It should be noted that Condran, Williams and Cheney in "Mortality in Philadelphia" find that water filtration had no effect on diarrheal deaths in this city. The experience of Philadelphia, however, appears to have been anomalous because studies of other cities such as Cincinnati, Boston, and Baltimore find that, as in Pittsburgh, water filtration helped significantly reduce infant deaths from diarrhea. For a review of other relevant historical studies, see Fuller, *Sewage Disposal*, pp. 101–24; van Poppel and van der Heijden, "A Review"; and Meckel, *Babies*, who presents evidence on the effects of Boston's public water and sewer system.

38. See Merrick, "Urban Brazil."

39. See Esrey, "A Multicountry Study" and Esrey, Habicht, and Casella, "Rural Lesotho."

40. See Brown, "Public Reform" and "Urban Environment." For a review of all of the historical and contemporary evidence on the relationship between infant mortality and public water and sewer systems, see van Poppel and van der Heijden, "A Review." See also, however, Lee, Rosenzweig, and Pitt, "High Mortality Populations," and Poskitt et al., "No Change in Growth."

41. See Watson, "Public Heath Investments" and Galiani, Gertler, and Schargrodsky, "Water for Life."

42. This problem could be addressed and the overall empirical analysis made much more revealing if the original manuscripts from this study could have been found. Unfortunately, an exhaustive search for the original manuscripts from this study (as well as other studies conducted by the Children's Bureau) suggests that the original, household-level responses have been lost or destroyed. The most recent effort to find the original Children's Bureau manuscripts was carried out at the National Archives under the auspices of the Center for Population Economics at the University of Chicago.

43. A household's race was determined by the nativity and ethnicity of the mother.

44. Household income was determined by the earnings of the father.

45. Condran and Preston in "Personal Health" show, for example, that infant mortality rates among French-Canadian immigrants to the United States were about three times greater than infant mortality rates among Jewish immigrants (171 per 1,000 live births versus 54 per 1,000). They attribute this differential to cultural differences in maternal feeding habits and labor force attachment. French-Canadian mothers returned to the labor force sooner and so were unable to breast-feed for as long a period as Jewish mothers.

Chapter 3

1. Cutler, Glaeser, and Vigdor, "American Ghetto," p. 466.

2. See Cutler, Glaeser, and Vigdor, "American Ghetto"; Massey and Denton, "Trends" and *American Apartheid*; Taeuber and Taeuber, *Negroes*; and White, "Segregation."

3. See Cutler, Glaeser, and Vigdor, "American Ghetto."

4. See Kellog, "Urban Clusters"; Russell, *Atlanta*; and Taeuber and Taeuber, *Negroes*, pp. 11–27.

5. Southern courts upheld these ordinances as constitutional as long as they did not require existing racial minorities on a particular street to move. See, for example, *Hopkins v. City of Richmond*, 117 Va. 692 (1915); *State of Maryland v. Gurry*, 121 Md. 534 (1913); and *Harris v. City of Louisville*, 177 S.W. 472 (1915). Although the U.S. Supreme Court eventually struck down all segregation ordinances as unconstitutional, southern cities continued to enact and enforce them. See Brophy *Dreamland*, pp. 84–85, and 154, notes 90–93.

6. For Woodward's argument, see *Strange Career*, p. 87. For the more recent econometric study, see Cutler, Glaeser, and Vigdor, "American Ghetto." For more current interpretations of the post-Reconstruction South, see Wright, *Old South*; and Ayers, *Promise*.

7. On the geographic fineness of housing segregation during the nineteenth century, see Cutler, Glaeser, and Vigdor, "American Ghetto" and Rabinowitz, *Race Relations*, pp. 107–11.

8. Kellog, "Urban Clusters."

9. See Waring, *Sewerage*.

10. See generally, Tarr, *Ultimate Sink*, pp. 173–74. On p. 174, table 6.1, Tarr reports that the urban population in the United States was 41.9 million, and estimates that between 34.7 and 41.8 million persons were connected to sewers. Tarr bases his estimates on various state and local sources.

11. Melosi's data on water come mainly from an article published in the *Journal of the American Water Works Assocation*. The data on sewers come from a report published by the U.S. Public Health Service in 1958. See Melosi, *Sanitary City*, p. 236.

12. As noted earlier, data are not available for cities with populations less than 30,000 and so the figure is restricted to cities with populations above that threshold.

13. See McNeill, *Plagues*, pp. 76–77 for a review and discussion of evidence.

14. See Beeson, DeJong, and Troesken, "Population Growth."

15. See U.S. Department of Labor, Children's Bureau, *Children of Preschool Age in Gary* and *Results of a Field Study in Baltimore*.

16. See U.S. Department of Labor, "Condition of the Negro."

17. The causes of this dramatic reduction are the subject of chapters 2, 4, and 6 of this book, and a larger related research project. For the moment, the goal is only to measure the extent to which the elimination of waterborne diseases contributed to increased longevity and reduced mortality. For a more general discussion of the decline in human mortality and its sources, see Fogel, "Nutrition" and Fogel and Costa, "Technophysio."

18. See, for example, Costa, "Understanding Decline."

19. See Linder and Grove, *Vital Statistics*, pp. 275–331.

20. See, generally, Hazen, *Clean Water* and Sedgwick and MacNutt, "Mills-Reincke Phenomenon." In *Drinking Water and Health*, the Commission on Life Sciences of the National Academy of Sciences recently concluded: "Even considering that typhoid is more likely

to be fatal than infectious hepatitis or gastroenteritis of unknown etiology, the Mills-Reincke theorem does seem to have considerable merit."

21. Koppes and Norris, "Ethnicity," p. 275.

22. See Preston and Haines, *Fatal Years*; Condran and Preston, "Personal Health"; and Ewbank and Preston, "Health Behavior."

23. The story told by Koppes and Norris is nearly identical to that developed by Preston and his collaborators, except that Koppes and Norris assume that the proper understanding of disease and household measures to prevent disease had been thoroughly disseminated among better-educated persons by 1900. The work of Preston and others suggests that it took another 20 years before such knowledge had been thoroughly learned and internalized by literate and well-educated parents.

24. North Carolina State Board of Health, *Biennial Report*, 1889, p. 156.

25. On the price of bottled water, see Florida State Board of Health, *Thirty-Second Report* 1920–1921, pp. 142–43. On the price of tap water, see U.S. Bureau of Census, *General Statistics of Cities*, 1915, pp. 159–70.

26. City of Memphis, *Artesian Water Plant*, pp. 108–09.

27. Curschmann, *Typhoid Fever*, pp. 43–65 and Whipple, *Typhoid*, pp. 1–6.

28. Florida State Board of Health, *Thirty-Second Report*, 1921–1922, pp. 152–53.

29. U.S. Bureau of Census, *Historical Statistics*, p. 382.

30. The econometric work in chapter 6 demonstrates that blacks gained more from water filtration than whites. In this chapter I am developing the argument that racial disparities in literacy rates help explain this differential effect. There is, however, an important caveat to this argument. The statistical work presented in Preston and Haines, *Fatal Years*, clearly shows that maternal literacy rates had a relatively small effect on child mortality in turn-of-the-century America, probably reducing child mortality rates by no more than 14 percent. In developing countries today, maternal literacy rates have a much larger effect, reducing child mortality by about 25 percent. See Preston and Haines, *Fatal Years*, pp. 201–202. See also Esrey and Habicht, "Maternal Literacy," who present evidence that maternal literacy altered the effects of toilets and piped water on infant mortality. In particular, using data from modern-day Malaysia, they find that the introduction of toilets had larger benefits for families with an illiterate mother than for those with literate mothers. They find the opposite result for piped water, which benefitted the literate more than the illiterate.

31. Koppes and Norris, "Ethnicity," p. 265.

32. Fishback, Haines, and Kantor, "New Deal."

33. For further data on Pittsburgh's sewer system, see chapter 4, table 4.1. The data in this paragraph are from the U.S. Census Bureau's *Social Statistics of Cities* and *General Statistics of Cities*, compiled by the Center for Population Economics, University of Chicago. See also Tarr, *Ultimate Sink*, pp. 90–94.

34. See Koppes and Norris, "Ethnicity."

35. The question emerges here of whether one should look at the percentage change, or the change in absolute levels. For example, in percentage terms, typhoid death rates for

blacks and native-born whites showed very similar changes, but in absolute terms, blacks experienced a much larger reduction in rates. This issue is thoroughly examined in chapter 7 and that analysis suggests that the absolute change (not the percentage change) is the appropriate metric.

36. Neighborhoods were much smaller geographic units than city wards.

37. Unfortunately, data on access to public water and sewer lines are available only at the neighborhood level, not the household level. Standard errors have been adjusted accordingly.

Chapter 4

1. For a comparison of death rates from different epidemics, see Wrenn, "A Reappraisal," pp. 5–6. Wrenn notes, however, that "During the 1878 epidemic, Memphis may have had the highest death rate ... from an epidemic of any city in the United States, but many cities have suffered from catastrophic epidemics."

2. Tennessee State Board of Health, *First Report*, pp. 105–06.

3. Hassell, *Memphis*, pp. 61–62.

4. In part because of repeated exposure over many generations, blacks had developed some innate resistence to both yellow fever and malaria. This issue is discussed and fully annotated with supporting sources in chapter 7.

5. See Tennessee State Board of Health, *First Report*, pp. 63–106.

6. See Hassell, *Memphis*, pp. 61–62 and Warner, "Hunting Yellow Fever."

7. See Pritchett and Tunali, "Strangers' Disease," and Tennessee State Board of Health, *First Report*, pp. 95–97. See also, Humphreys, *Yellow Fever*.

8. See Tennessee State Board of Health, *First Report*, pp. 95–97.

9. Savannah, *Report of the Mayor*, p. 161.

10. See Mokyr, "Why More Work?" and Tomes, *Gospel of Germs*, pp. 78–91.

11. On the possibility of transferring yellow fever through such articles, see Tennessee State Board of Health, *First Report*, pp. 95–96. The subsequent development of the germ theory of disease might have undermined the idea that climate affected diseases, but it did little to quell the fear of dirt and unsanitary living conditions, or the fear that diseases could spread easily from the poor to the wealthy. See generally, Mokyr, "Why More Work?" and Tomes, *Gospel of Germs*.

12. The quotation is from Ellis, "Sanitary Revolution." Other data and information are from Ellis, *Yellow Fever*, pp. 112–13.

13. See Hassell, *Memphis*, pp. 61–68 and Tennessee State Board of Health, *First Report*, pp. 83–109 and 319–27.

14. On the bankruptcy of Memphis following the epidemic, see Bejach, "Taxing District"; Ellis, "Disease" and "Sanitary Revolution"; and Wrenn, "A Reappraisal" and "Sewer Experiment." On the growth of the city before and after the epidemic, see Capers, *River Town*, pp. 75–89 and Miller, *Memphis*, pp. 50–51.

15. Cassedy, "Colonel Waring"; Tarr, *Ultimate Sink*, pp. 131–58; and Waring, *Sewerage*.

16. See Wrenn, "Sewer Experiment" and Waring, *Sewerage*, pp. 114–23.

17. Memphis *Daily Appeal*, December 11, 1879, p. 4.

18. Memphis *Daily Appeal*, December 11, 1879, p. 4.

19. Memphis *Daily Appeal*, January 11, 1880, p. 1.

20. Elliot, *Memphis Sewer System*, pp. 11–12.

21. These calculations are based on data from Elliot, *Memphis Sewer System*, pp. 25–27.

22. Tennessee State Board of Health, *First Report*, pp. 328–30.

23. A more precise map is available upon request.

24. See, for example, Ellis, *Yellow Fever*, pp. 113–15 and Wrenn, "Sewer Experiment."

25. When the city annexed large portions of neighboring land in 1899, the proportion of households with service fell sharply, but recovered to high levels of service within a decade. See Miller, *Memphis*, pp. 50–51 and U.S. Bureau of Census, *General Statistics of Cities*, 1909, pp. 86–92.

26. Savannah, *Report of the Mayor*, pp. 1–16.

27. Another potential explanation for the differences observed across Memphis and Savannah focuses on the question of timing. Memphis first built its sewer system during the early 1880s, just after Reconstruction, while Savannah did not build its sewer system until 1900. It is well known that blacks became increasingly disenfranchised and politically impotent over the course of the nineteenth and early twentieth centuries; things got worse, not better, as time progressed. See Margo, *Race and Schooling*, pp. 18–24; Ayers, *Promise*; and Willis, *Forgotten Time*.

28. As with Memphis, this map does not replicate the exact location of sewer mains or households. Rather it has been constructed to maximize readability and is intended only to convey the broad contours of the sewer system and the location of different racial groups. A more precise map is available from the author upon request.

29. Federal Writer's Project, *Savannah*, p. 118.

30. U.S. Department of Labor, "Condition of Negro," pp. 260–61.

31. The history and location of these sites are from FWP, pp. 48–52. For the history and current status of the First Bryan Baptist Church and the Laurel Grove South Cemetery, see the following website: http://www.soulofamerica.com/cityfldr/savannah2.html. Regarding the public school in Yamacraw, according to the FWP (p. 51): "In 1878, the Board of Education established its first public school for Negroes, and through Mr. DeRenne [who donated the land and building] the old Scarborough Mansion was secured. It is located in Yamacraw."

32. These data are from Cutler, Glaeser, and Vigdor, "American Ghetto."

33. Terry, "The Negro," p. 300.

34. Terry, "The Negro," p. 304.

35. Terry, "The Negro," p. 304.

36. Terry, "The Negro," p. 306.

37. Terry, "Extermination," pp. 14–15.

38. Terry, "Extermination," p. 15.

39. Terry, "Extermination," p. 16.

40. Terry, "Extermination," p. 16.

41. Terry, "Extermination," p. 15.

42. Terry, "The Negro," p. 309.

43. Terry wrote: "[I]t must be remembered that if we condemn every house that is unfit for habitation in Jacksonville, we would condemn 33 percent of all our houses, and that 90 percent of these are occupied by negroes. Now a house not connected with a sewer and city water supply would be admitted by most to be unfit for habitation, but our sewerage system does not cover more than two-thirds of the population at the most.... [I]n the negro district ... the open privy (now screened but still a privy) is in use, [and] the number of families residing to a block far exceeds those residing in the sewered district.... As soon as we discover any house in a sewered district not connected with a sewer, we condemn it, but we cannot touch the non-sewered district by any such method." Terry, "The Negro," p. 309.

44. See the appendix, particularly table A.1, for further a complete analysis of the sewer data from the Negro Mortality Project (including the data on Jacksonville) and a thorough discussion of its compilation and findings.

45. U.S. Bureau of Census, *General Statistics of Cities*, 1909.

46. The Jacksonville death rate from typhoid fever (155 deaths per 100,000) is an adjusted figure and much higher than the original figure (93.1) stated in the official mortality statistics. The adjusted figure reflects the fact that typhoid was often underdiagnosed in the American South because doctors tended to confuse typhoid with malaria. Chapter 7 fully explains and justifies the use of the "malaria-adjusted" typhoid rate (see in particular, section 7.5). Nevertheless, even if one prefers the original data reported by government officials, Jacksonville's typhoid rate still appears to have been inordinately high. The average reported death rate from typhoid in Jacksonville between 1906 and 1910 was 93.1, 3.5 times the national average. See U.S. Bureau of Census, *Mortality Statistics*, 1910, pp. 27–30.

47. Terry, "Extermination," pp. 14–15.

48. Terry, "Extermination," p. 15.

49. Tarr, *Ultimate Sink*, p. 93.

50. Terry, "The Negro," p. 304.

51. Terry, "The Negro," p. 303.

52. Terry, "The Negro," pp. 300–01.

53. Brunner "Negro Health," p. 186.

54. Brunner "Negro Health," p. 187.

55. Brunner "Negro Health," p. 188.

56. All of the quotations are from, Brunner, "Negro Health," p. 183.

57. Brunner, "Negro Health," p. 184.

Chapter 5

1. For the basic facts of the case, see *Hawkins v. Town of Shaw, Mississippi*, 437 F. 2d 1286 (1971).

2. Graham and Kravitt, "Evolution of Equal Protection," p. 108.

3. Simon, "Equal Protection," p. 498.

4. Reflections on the current state of public services can be found in McNulty, "Twenty Years Later." A civil rights activist during the 1960s, and a Presbyterian minister, McNulty provides a detailed firsthand account of conditions in Shaw 20 years after he first saw the town during his work for civil rights legislation and reform. On access to public water and sewer lines in Shaw, see http://www.amshomefinder.com/MS/MS011013630.html.

5. For data on death rates, see U.S. Bureau of Census, *Census*, 1900 and *Mortality Statistics*, 1920; and Linder and Grove, *Vital Statistics*.

6. All quotations and historical observations in this paragraph are from Ayers, *Promise*, pp. 194–95. On the rise of delta region, see generally Willis, *Forgotten Time*, pp. 5–80, and Irwin and O'Brien "Economic Progress."

7. The sources of information for this paragraph are *Hawkins v. Town of Shaw*, 437 F. 2d 1286 (1971); *Hawkins v. Town of Shaw*, 303 F. Supp. 1162 (1969); and U.S. Bureau of Census, *Census*, 1970. See also Willis, *Forgotten Time*.

8. See Willis, *Forgotten Time*, pp. 114–86.

9. All data are from the U.S. Bureau of Census, *Census*, 1970.

10. *Hawkins v. Town of Shaw*, 437 F. 2d 1286 (1971), p. 1291.

11. *Hawkins v. Town of Shaw*, 437 F. 2d 1286 (1971). For additional details, see also *Hawkins v. Town of Shaw*, 303 F. Supp. 1162 (1969).

12. *Hawkins v. Town of Shaw*, 437 F. 2d 1286 (1971), p. 1289.

13. Some legal commentators, however, argue that *Shaw* is important because it deals with issues analogous to those advanced by environmental activists who believe the siting of landfills and other dangerous economic activities is racially biased. See, for example, Hill and Targ, "Environmental Justice."

14. *Dowdell et al. v. Apopka* 698 F. 2d 1181 (1983), p. 1183. The role of segregation ordinances in giving rise to residential segregation is discussed in chapter 3.

15. See *Dobson et al. v. Dade City* 594 F. Supp. 1274 (1984), pp. 1275–77.

16. *Johnson v. City of Arcadia* 450 F. Supp. 1363 (1978), p. 1365.

17. *Kennedy Park Homes Association v. City of Lackawanna* 436 F. 2d 108 (1970), p. 109.

18. See *Hadnott v. City of Prattville* 309 F. Supp. 967 (1970). See also Tarr, *Ultimate Sink*, pp. 90–1.

19. Ruggles and Sobek, *Integrated Public Use Micro Data Series*, hereafter cited as IPUMS.

Chapter 6

1. This interregional variation might reflect the fact that blacks who died from typhoid were more likely to have been misdiagnosed with malaria in the South than in the non-South, where malaria was much less common. No adjustments have been made to the data here for this potential underreporting of typhoid. As shown in chapter 7, this biases the estimation against finding any effect of filtration, and makes it more likely to find evidence that African Americans had relatively limited access to public water supplies.

2. Nevertheless, to control for the possibility that cities that installed filters differed in some systematic and time-varying manner from cities that did not, city-specific time trends were added to the regressions. See also Troesken, "Typhoid."

3. The fact that the difference and the ratio yield conflicting results is important and is explored fully in chapter 7.

4. In chapter 7 I explain why the difference is preferable to the ratio as a measure of inequitable access to public water and sewer lines.

5. This sensitivity is important and is fully explored in chapter 7.

6. For details about the precise construction of this index, see Cutler, Glaeser, and Vigdor, "American Ghetto."

7. Again, it is worth noting that the difference and the ratio yield inconsistent findings; this issue is discussed in chapter 7.

Chapter 7

1. See examples presented in chapter 2 and Galishoff, *Newark*, pp. 185–87; McCarthy, *Philadelphia*, pp. 5–40; Meeker, "Social Return"; Tarr, *Ultimate Sink*, pp. 90–92; Melosi, *Sanitary City*, pp. 136–49; Wing, "Typhoid"; and Fuller, "Water-Works."

2. See Mokyr, "Why More Work?"; Mokyr and Stein, "Science"; and Tomes, *Gospel of Germs*. Mokyr and Tomes establish the plausibility of the hypothesis that private investments in health mattered. But the strongest evidence for this hypothesis can be found in Condran and Preston, "Personal Health"; Ewbank and Preston, "Health Behavior"; and Preston and Haines, *Fatal Years*, pp. 200–210.

3. This wavelike pattern is not unique to typhoid but is observed for most infectious diseases. As McNeill explains in his classic work, *Plagues and Peoples* (p. 77), "As the local supply of susceptible hosts runs out, the infection dies and disappears, except in the urban center whence it originally emerged. There, enough susceptibles will remain for the infectious organism to keep itself alive until disease experienced individuals again accumulate . . . and another epidemic flare-up becomes a possibility."

4. See Meeker, "Social Return."

5. See, for example, Ellis, *Yellow Fever*; Russell, *Atlanta* and "Municipal Services"; Galishoff, "Germs"; and Hoffman, "Progressive Public Health."

6. Doyle, *New Men*, p. 283.

7. See figure 10.4, p. 282 in Doyle's *New Men*.

8. Studies using ratios include Ewbank, "Black Mortality" and Doyle, *New Men*, pp. 282–83. Studies using differences include Troesken, "Race." These studies do not discuss why one metric is preferable to another.

9. One objection to this model is that it imposes a linear relationship on typhoid rates and bacteria. Clearly, however, in practice it is a simple matter to transform the data to allow for a nonlinear relationship. For example, in the empirical work described here I use the natural log of bacteria.

10. See, for example, Ewbank's well-known article "Black Mortality," on black-white differences in mortality, particularly differences in typhoid rates. The same is true of my article, "Race."

11. See North Carolina State Board of Health, *Biennial Report*.

12. Terry, "The Negro," p. 303.

13. *The Cambridge World History of Human Disease*, edited by Kenneth F. Kiple, contains extensive discussions of malaria and black resistance to that disease. See pp. 39, 294–95, 448–50, 526–27, and 855–62. A shorter explanation can be found in McNeill, *Plagues* who writes (p. 66): "African cultivators were nevertheless able to persist in their effort to tame the rain forest for agriculture; not, however, without genetic adaption whereby the frequency of a gene that produces sickle-shaped red corpuscles in heterozygous individuals increased markedly. Such cells are less hospitable to the malarial plasmodium than normal red blood cells. Consequently, the debilitating effects of malarial infection are reduced in individuals who have this kind of red corpuscle. But the cost of such protection was very high. Individuals who inherit the sickling gene from both parents die young." On the role that natural selection might have also played in promoting innate immunities to disease, see Lee, "Socioeconomic Background." See also Warren, "Northern Chills," who discusses of the role that disease immunities (and vulnerabilities) played in determining the geographic location of slavery and black populations in the United States; and Humphreys, who in *Malaria* explores the social context of malaria in the American South.

14. See, however, Humphreys, *Malaria*, who argues that malaria was highly correlated with poverty and substandard housing in the turn-of-the-century South.

15. The history of Jacksonville is fully described and annotated in chapter 4.

16. From the annual report of the Richmond health department, quoted in U.S. Bureau of Census, *Mortality Statistics*, 1910, pp. 27–28.

17. It is notable that for blacks and whites, malaria rates fell sharply after 1909. Why did this happen? Two forces were at work. First, around this time, the Richmond health department approached the aforementioned three doctors who were attributing deaths to malaria at unusually high rates and requested that they reexamine their diagnostic techniques. The health department also began investigating and verifying all deaths reported as malaria. See U.S. Bureau of Census, *Mortality Statistics*, 1910, pp. 27–28. Second, the city installed a water filter in 1909. Filtration reduced the number of true cases of typhoid and therefore also reduced the number of cases of typhoid falsely diagnosed as malaria. U.S. Bureau of Census, *General Statistics of Cities*, 1915.

18. In a recent paper in the *Journal of Social History*, Steven Hoffman describes black and white typhoid rates in Richmond (pp. 179–180): "In a city where African Americans died at almost twice the rate of whites, typhoid fever was one of the few diseases that afflicted whites more often than blacks. Between 1900 and 1910, only in one year, 1904, did more blacks die of the disease than whites.... In a city plagued by a significantly higher African-American death rate almost across the board, typhoid fever was a notable exception." Hoffman offers no explanation for this exceptional finding, but nevertheless proceeds to use these same data as evidence that blacks were discriminated against in the provision of public health. The findings here suggest that black typhoid rates were underreported and misdiagnosed as malaria. See Hoffman, "Progressive Public Health."

19. These findings prompt the question of why blacks were more likely than whites to have had their illness diagnosed incorrectly. One plausible answer is that whites could afford better health care, including increased access to Widal tests (the definitive method of diagnosing typhoid). Because blacks had fewer financial resources than whites, they often would have had to forgo medical care and when they got care, they probably could not afford a Widal test. For a further discussion of this general issue, see chapter 3.

Chapter 8

1. For the moment, set aside concerns about the potential simultaneity between growth in mains and population growth. This issue is addressed later.

2. Small sample sizes make it impossible to apply this procedure to the 1908 and 1911 data.

3. These results can also be stated in terms of the hypotheses outlined earlier. The results for segregated cities are consistent with hypothesis 8.1 and the results for integrated cities are consistent with hypothesis 8.3.

4. Another possibility is that these cross-sectional data employ different samples of cities than those used in the analysis of panel data.

5. All values are in levels, not logs. With a logarithmic specification, the coefficients would measure elasticities, which are not useful statistics for the question at hand. Because blacks represented a much smaller fraction of the population than whites, providing service to a 10 percent increase in the black population would have required a much smaller extension in the system of mains than a 10 percent increase in the white population would have.

6. The fact that the 1890–1900 sample and the 1900–1920 sample yield different conclusions is unsettling and might be caused by the fact that the regional composition of the samples varies. The earlier sample employs data for southern cities and towns exclusively, while the later sample employs data for large cities across the United States.

Chapter 9

1. See Koppes and Norris, "Ethncity."

2. See Cutler, Glaeser, and Vigdor, "American Ghetto."

3. See Doyle, *New Men*, pp. 281–84.

4. In a response to one of Dr. Terry's papers, a doctor affiliated with the U.S. Public Health Service, L. L. Lumsden, argued that extending water and sewer lines was a good idea because it would drive up property values in black neighborhoods and in turn drive blacks out of urban environments into the country, where, Lumsden believed, blacks belonged and where their diseases could not spread to white households. See Terry, "The Negro," p. 307.

5. See Meeker, "Social Return," for an estimate of the returns to investments in public health.

6. Higgs, *Competition*, pp. 22–23.

7. See Roback, "Street Cars" and Fishback, *Soft Coal*, pp. 184–90.

8. See McKeown, *Modern Population* and Fogel, "Nutrition."

9. See Szreter, "Economic Growth" and "Social Intervention."

Appendix

1. U.S. Department of Labor, "Condition of the Negro."

2. U.S. Department of Labor, "Condition of the Negro," p. 258.

3. U.S. Department of Labor, "Condition of the Negro," p. 258; "cluster" is inserted for clarity.

4. U.S. Department of Labor, "Condition of the Negro," p. 258. Italics added.

5. All of the statistics on access to public water and sewer lines are based on questions that investigators asked about the presence of bathrooms and/or water closets in households. I assume that all households with bathrooms and/or water closets were connected to both public water and sewer lines. This assumption understates access to public water because households frequently had water spigots and faucets serviced by public water mains but at the same time did not have bathrooms and water closets. This assumption also overstates access to public sewers because households sometimes used toilets and water closets without connecting to public sewers, despite the fact that city officials tried their best to discourage this practice. I base this discussion on personal communications with Joel Tarr of Carnegie Mellon University.

6. See U.S. Bureau of Census, *Historical Statistics*, pp. 320–26 for aggregated data on family size. See also U.S. Department of Labor, "Condition of the Negro," for data on the size of African-American families around the same time.

References

Adu, D., Y. Anim-Addo, A. K. Foli, E. D. Yeboah, and J. K. Quartey. 1975. "Acute Renal Failure and Typhoid Fever." *Ghana Medical Journal*, 14: 172–74.

Ali, Gazanfar, Samia Rashid, M. A. Kamli, Parvez A. Shah, and G. Q. Allaqaband. 1997. "Spectrum of Neuropsychiatric Complications in 791 Cases of Typhoid Fever." *Tropical Medicine and International Health*, 2: 314–18.

American City (magazine). No author. 1920 and 1921 issues.

American Water Works Association. 1926. *Water Works Practice: A Manual*. Baltimore, Md.: Williams and Wilkins.

Armstrong, Gregory L., Laura A. Conn, and Robert W. Pinner. 1999. "Trends in Infectious Disease Mortality in the United States During the 20th Century." *Journal of the American Medical Association*, 281: 61–66.

Ayers, Edward. 1992. *The Promise of the New South: Life After Reconstruction*. New York: Oxford University Press.

Baker, Moses N. 1897. *The Manual of American Waterworks*. New York: Engineering News Press.

Beardsley, Edward H. 1987. *A History of Neglect: Health Care for Blacks and Mill Workers in the Twentieth-Century South*. Knoxville: University of Tennessee Press.

Beeson, Patricia E., David N. DeJong, and Werner Troesken. 2001. "Population Growth in U.S. Counties, 1840–1990." *Regional Science and Urban Economics*, 31: 669–99.

Bejach, L. D. 1948. "The Taxing District of Shelby County." *West Tennessee Historical Society Papers*, 2: 1–27.

Blake, Nelson. 1956. *Water for the Cities: A History of the Urban Water Supply Problem in the United States*. Syracuse, N.Y.: Syracuse University Press.

Brophy, Alfred L. 2002. *Reconstructing the Dreamland: The Tulsa Race Riot of 1921: Race, Reparations, and Reconciliation*. New York: Oxford University Press.

Brown, John C. 1989. "Public Reform or Private Gain? The Case of Investments in Sanitary Infrastructure: Germany, 1880–1887." *Urban Studies*, 26: 2–12.

Brown, John C. 1989. "Reforming the Urban Environment: Sanitation, Housing, and Government Intervention in Germany, 1870–1910." *Journal of Economic History*, 49: 450–72.

Brundage, W. Fitzhugh. 1993. *Lynching in the New South: Georgia and Virginia*. Urbana: University of Illinois Press.

Brunner, William F. 1913. "The Negro Health Problem in Southern Cities." *American Journal of Public Health*, 5: 183–190.

Buck, C., and H. Simpson. 1982. "Infant Diarrhoea and Subsequent Mortality from Heart Disease and Cancer." *Journal of Epidemiology and Community Health*, 36: 27–30.

Budd, William. 1873. "Typhoid Fever: Its Nature, Mode of Spreading, and Prevention." Reprinted in *American Journal of Public Health*, 8: 610–12.

Cain, Louis P., and Elyce J. Rotella. 2001. "Death and Spending: Urban Mortality and Municipal Expenditure on Sanitation." *Annales de Démographie Historique*, 45: 139–54.

Capers, Gerald M. 1939. *The Biography of a River Town, Memphis: Its Heroic Age*. Chapel Hill: University of North Carolina Press.

Cassedy, James H. 1962. "The Flamboyant Colonel Waring: An Anti-Contagionist Holds the American Stage in the Age of Pasteur and Koch." *Bulletin of the History of Medicine*, 36: 163–76.

Collins, William J., and Robert A. Margo. 2001. "Race and Home Ownership: A Century-Long View." *Explorations in Economic History*, 38: 68–92.

Condran, Gretchen A., and Ellen Crimmins-Gardner. 1978. "Public Health Measures and Mortality in U.S. Cities in the Late Nineteenth Century." *Human Ecology*, 6: 27–54.

Condran, Gretchen A., and Samuel H. Preston. 1994. "Child Mortality Differences, Personal Health Care Practices, and Medical Technology: The United States, 1900–30." In *Health and Social Change in International Perspective*, Lincoln C. Chen, Arthur Kleinman, and N. C. Ware, Eds. Harvard Series on Population and International Health. Boston: Harvard University Press.

Condran, Gretchen A., H. Williams, and R. A. Cheney. 1984. "The Decline in Mortality in Philadelphia from 1870 to 1930: The Role of Municipal Services." *Pennsylvania Magazine of History and Biography*, 108: 153–77.

Costa, Dora L. 2000. "Understanding the Twentieth-Century Decline in Chronic Conditions among Older Men." *Demography*, 37: 53–72.

Costa, Dora L. 2003. "Understanding Mid-Life and Older Age Mortality Declines: Evidence from the Union-Army Veterans." *Journal of Econometrics*, 112: 175–92.

Curschmann, H. 1901. *Typhoid Fever and Typhus Fever*. Philadelphia: W. B. Saunders.

Cutler, David M., Edward L. Glaeser, and Jacob L. Vigdor. 1999. "The Rise and Decline of the American Ghetto." *Journal of Political Economy*, 107: 455–506.

Donohue, John H. III, and James Heckman. 1991. "Continuous versus Episodic Change: The Impact of Civil Rights Policy on the Economic Status of Blacks." *Journal of Economic Literature*, 29: 1603–43.

Doyle, Don H. 1990. *New Men, New Cities, New South: Atlanta, Nashville, Charleston, Mobile, 1860–1910*. Chapel Hill: University of North Carolina Press.

Elliot, James H. 1891. *A Description of the Memphis Sewer System, 1879 to 1890, Inclusive*. Memphis: Press of S. C. Toof & Co.

Ellis, John H. 1964. "Memphis' Sanitary Revolution, 1880–1890." *Tennessee Historical Quarterly*, 23: 59–72.

Ellis, John H. 1974. "Disease and the Destiny of a City: The 1878 Yellow Fever Epidemic in Memphis." *West Tennessee Historical Society Papers*, 38: 75–89.

Ellis, John H. 1992. *Yellow Fever and Public Health in the New South*. Lexington: University of Kentucky Press.

Ellms, Joseph W. 1913. "Disinfection of Public Water Supplies: Why the Purification of Drinking Water Should Be Supplemented by Disinfection—the Uses of Chlorine, Ozone, and Ultra-Violet Light." *American City*, 22: 564–68.

Elo, Irma T., and Samuel H. Preston. 1994. "Estimating African-American Mortality from Inaccurate Data." *Demography*, 33: 427–58.

Esrey, S. A. 1996. "Water, Waste, and Well-Being: A Multicountry Study." *American Journal of Epidemiology*, 143: 608–23.

Esrey, S. A., and J. P. Habicht. 1988. "Maternal Literacy Modifies the Effect of Toilets and Piped Water on Infant Survival in Malaysia." *American Journal of Epidemiology*, 127: 1079–87.

Esrey, S. A., J. P. Habicht, and G. Casella. 1992. "The Complementary Effect of Latrines and Increased Water Usage on the Growth of Infants in Rural Lesotho." *American Journal of Epidemiology*, 135: 659–66.

Ewbank, Douglas C. 1987. "History of Black Mortality and Health before 1940." *Milbank Quarterly*, 65(Suppl. 1): 101–28.

Ewbank, Douglas C., and Samuel H. Preston. 1990. "Personal Health Behavior and the Decline in Infant and Child Mortality: The United States, 1900–1930." In *What We Know about Health Transition: The Cultural, Social, and Behavioral Determinants of Health*, John Caldwell, Sally Findley, Pat Caldwell, Gigi Santow, Wendy Cosford, Jennifer Braid and Daphne Broers-Freeman, Eds. Health Transition Center, Canberra: Australian National University.

Federal Writers' Project. Savannah Unit. 1937. *Savannah*. Savannah, Ga.: Review Printing Company.

Fergerson, Gerard. 1994. "To Live Poor but Healthy: Typhoid and the Politics of Public Health in Boston, 1880–1920." Unpublished doctoral dissertation. Department of the History of Science. Harvard University.

Fishback, Price. 1989. *Soft Coal, Hard Choices: The Economic Welfare of Bituminous Coal Miners, 1890–1930*. New York: Oxford University Press.

Fishback, Price, Michael Haines, and Shawn Kantor. 2000. "The Impact of New Deal Programs on Black and White Infant Mortality in the South." *Explorations in Economic History*, 38: 93–122.

Florida State Board of Health. *Report of the State Board of Health*. Jacksonville, Fla.: The Palatka News. Various years, 1914–1922.

Fogel, Robert W. 1986. "Nutrition and the Decline in Mortality since 1700: Some Preliminary Findings." In *Long-Term Factors in American Economic Growth*, Stanley L. Engerman and Robert E. Gallman, Eds., pp. 439–556. Chicago: University of Chicago Press.

Fogel, Robert W. 1989. *Without Consent or Contract: The Rise and Fall of American Slavery.* New York: Norton.

Fogel, Robert W., and Dora L. Costa. 1997. "A Theory of Technophysio Evolution, with Some Implications for Forecasting Population, Health Care Costs, and Pension Costs." *Demography,* 34: 49–66.

Fuller, George W. 1912. *Sewage Disposal.* New York: McGraw-Hill.

Fuller, George W. 1928. "Water-Works in the United States." *Transactions of the American Society of Civil Engineers,* 92: 1209–1224.

Gadgil, Ashok. 1998. "Drinking Water in Developing Countries." *Annual Review of Energy and the Environment,* 23: 253–86.

Galiani, Sebastian, Paul Gertler, and Ernesto Schargrodsky. 2003. "Water for Life: The Impact of the Privatization of Water Services on Child Mortality." Paper presented at the BREAD (Bureau for Research in Economic Analysis of Development) Conference, February 7 and 8, 2003. Washington, D.C.

Galishoff, Stuart. 1985. "Germs Know No Color Line: Black Health and Public Policy in Atlanta, 1900–1918." *Journal of the History of Medicine,* 40: 22–41.

Galishoff, Stuart. 1988. *Newark: The Nation's Unhealthiest City, 1832–1895.* New Brunswick, N.J.: Rutgers University Press.

Graham, Robert L., and Jason H. Kravitt. 1972. "The Evolution of Equal Protection— Education, Municipal Services, and Wealth." *Harvard Civil Rights-Civil Liberties Law Review,* 7: 105–99.

Haines, Michael R. 1994. "Estimated Life Tables for the United States, 1850–1900." Historical Paper No. 59. Cambridge, Mass.: National Bureau of Economic Research.

Haines, Michael R. 2001. "The Urban Mortality Transition in the United States, 1800–1940." Historical Paper No. 134. Cambridge, Mass.: National Bureau of Economic Research.

Haines, Michael R. 2002. "Ethnic Differences in Demographic Behavior in the United States: Has There Been Convergence?" Working Paper 9042. Cambridge, Mass.: National Bureau of Economic Research. (Available at http://www.nber.org/papers/w9042.)

Hassell, Joan. 1982. *Memphis, 1800–1900.* Vol. III. *Years of Courage, 1870–1900.* New York: Nancy Powers.

Hazen, Allen. 1907. *Clean Water and How to Get It.* New York: Wiley.

Higgs, Robert. 1979. "Cycles and Trends of Mortality in 18 Large American Cities, 1871–1900." *Explorations in Economic History,* 16: 381–408.

Higgs, Robert. 1980. *Competition and Coercion: Blacks in the American Economy, 1865–1914.* Chicago: University of Chicago Press.

Higgs, Robert. 1982. "Accumulation of Property by Southern Blacks before World War I." *American Economic Review,* 72: 725–37.

Higgs, Robert, and Douglas Booth. 1979. "Mortality Differentials within Large American Cities in 1890." *Human Ecology,* 7: 353–70.

Hill, Barry E., and Nicholas Targ. 2000. "The Link between Protecting Natural Resources and the Issue of Environmental Justice." *Boston College Environmental Affairs Legal Review*, 28: 1–122.

Hoffman, Steven J. 2001. "Progressive Public Health Administration in the Jim Crow South: A Case Study of Richmond, Virginia, 1907–1920." *Journal of Social History*, 35: 177–94.

Humphreys, Margaret. 1992. *Yellow Fever and the South*. New Brunswick, N.J.: Rutgers University Press.

Humphreys, Margaret. 2003. *Malaria: Poverty, Race, and Public Health in the United States*. Baltimore, Md.: Johns Hopkins University Press.

Irwin, James R., and Anthony Patrick O'Brien. 2001. "Economic Progress in the Postbellum South? African-American Incomes in the Mississippi Delta, 1880–1910." *Explorations in Economic History*, 38: 166–80.

Kant Panday, Chandra, Namita Singh, Vijay Kumar, Anil Agarwal, and Prabhat Kumar Singh. 2002. "Typhoid, Hepatitis E, or Typhoid and Hepatitis E: The Cause of Fulminant Hepatic Failure—A Diagnostic Dilemma." *Critical Care Medicine*, 20: 376–78.

Kellog, John. 1977. "Negro Urban Clusters in the Postbellum South." *Geographical Review*, 67: 310–21.

Khosla, S. N. 1981. "The Heart in Enteric (Typhoid) Fever." *Journal of Tropical Medicine and Hygiene*, 84: 125–31.

Khosla, S. N. 1990. "Typhoid Hepatitis." *Postgraduate Medical Journal*, 66: 923–25.

Khosla, S. N., and R. Lochan. 1992. "Renal Dysfunction in Enteric Fever." *Journal of the Association of Physicians of India*, 39: 382–84.

Kiple, Kenneth F. 1993. *The Cambridge World History of Human Disease*. Cambridge: Cambridge University Press.

Koppes, Clayton R., and William P. Norris. 1985. "Ethnicity, Class, and Mortality in the Industrial City: A Case Study of Typhoid Fever in Pittsburgh, 1890–1910." *Journal of Urban History*, 11: 259–79.

Le, V. D., Q. Y. Tran, V. C. Nguyen, T. N. Nguyen, and K. C. Tran. 1976. "Typhoid Fever with Hepatitis." *Journal of Tropical Medicine and Hygiene*, 79: 25–7.

Leavitt, Judith Walzer. 1996. *Typhoid Mary: Captive to the Public's Health*. Boston: Beacon Press.

Lee, Chulhee. 1997. "Socioeconomic Background, Disease, and Mortality among Union Army Recruits: Implications for Economic and Demographic History." *Explorations in Economic History*, 34: 27–55.

Lee, Lung-fei, Mark R. Rosenzweig, and Mark M. Pitt. 1997. "The Effects of Improved Nutrition, Sanitation, and Water Quality on Child Health in High-Mortality Populations." *Journal of Econometrics*, 77: 209–35.

Levy, Ernest C., and W. T. Tuck. 1913. "The Maggot Trap—A New Weapon in Our Warfare against the Typhoid Fly." *American Journal of Public Health*, 3: 657–60.

Linder, Forrest E., and Robert D. Grove. 1943. *Vital Statistics Rates in the United States, 1900–1940*. U.S. Department of Commerce. Bureau of the Census. Washington, D.C.: Government Printing Office.

Lindholt, J. S., H. Fasting, E. W. Henneberg, and L. Ostergaard. 1999. "A Review of *Chlamydia* Pneumonia and Atherosclerosis." *European Journal of Vascular and Endovascular Surgery*, 17: 283–89.

Lineberry, Robert L. 1977. *Equality and Urban Policy: The Distribution of Municipal Public Services*. Beverly Hills, Calif.: Sage.

Margo, Robert A. 1984. "Accumulation of Property by Southern Blacks before World War One: Comment and Further Evidence." *American Economic Review*, 74: 768–76.

Margo, Robert A. 1990. *Race and Schooling in the South, 1880–1950: An Economic History*. Chicago: University of Chicago Press.

Markel, Howard. 1995. "'Knocking Out the Cholera': Cholera, Class, and Quarantines in New York City, 1892." *Bulletin of the History of Medicine*, 69: 420–57.

Massey, Douglas S., and Nancy A. Denton. 1987. "Trends in the Residential Segregation of Blacks, Hispanics, and Asians: 1970–1980." *American Sociological Review*, 94: 802–25.

Massey, Douglas S., and Nancy A. Denton. 1993. *American Apartheid: Segregation and the Making of the Underclass*. Cambridge, Mass.: Harvard University Press.

Mathai, Elizabeth, T. Jacob John, Mallika Rani et al. 1995. "Significance of *Salmonella typhi* Bacteriuria." *Journal of Clinical Microbiology*, 33: 1791–92.

McCarthy, Michael P. 1987. *Typhoid and the Politics of Public Health in Nineteenth-Century Philadelphia*. Philadelphia: American Philosophical Society.

McGraw Directory of American Water Companies, The. No author. 1917. New York: McGraw Publishing.

McKeown, Thomas J. 1976. *The Modern Rise of Population*. New York: Academic Press.

McNeill, William H. 1977. *Plagues and Peoples*. New York: Anchor Books, Doubleday.

McNulty, Edward. 1984. "The Mississippi Freedom Summer Twenty Years Later." Accessed on-line at Religion Online, at the following address: http://www.religion-online.org. The article originally appeared in the *Christian Century*, October 17, 1984, p. 959.

Meckel, Richard A. 1990. *Save the Babies: American Public Health Reform and the Prevention of Infant Mortality, 1850–1929*. Baltimore, Md.: Johns Hopkins University Press.

Meeker, Edward. 1974. "The Social Rate of Return on Investment in Public Health, 1880–1910." *Journal of Economic History*, 34: 392–421.

Melosi, Martin V. 2000. *The Sanitary City: Urban Infrastructure in America from Colonial Times to the Present*. Baltimore, Md.: Johns Hopkins University Press.

Memphis, City of. 1904. *Transcript of all the Proceedings of the [Memphis] Legislative Council of the City of Memphis Respecting the Purchase of the Artesian Water Plant*. Memphis: Press of S. C. Toof & Co.

Memphis *Daily Appeal*. Various issues, 1879–1880.

Merrick, Thomas W. 1985. "The Effect of Piped Water on Early Childhood Mortality in Urban Brazil, 1970 to 1976." *Demography*, 22: 1–24.

Miller, William D. 1957. *Memphis during the Progressive Era, 1900–1917.* Memphis, Tenn.: Memphis State University Press.

Mills, Hiram F. 1891. "Typhoid Fever in its Relation to Water-Supplies." *Journal of the New England Water Works Association*, 5: 149–61.

Mokyr, Joel. 2000. "Why 'More Work for Mother?' Knowledge and Household Behavior, 1870–1945." *Journal of Economic History*, 60: 1–41.

Mokyr, Joel, and Rebecca Stein. 1997. "Science, Health, and Household Technology: The Effect of the Pasteur Revolution on Consumer Demand." In *The Economics of New Goods*, Timothy F. Bresnahan and Robert J. Gordon, Eds. Chicago: University of Chicago Press.

Morgenstern, R., and P. C. Hayes. 1991. "The Liver in Typhoid Fever: Always Affected, Not Just a Complication." *American Journal of Gastroenterology*, 86: 1235–39.

Murray, Charles. 1984. *Losing Ground: American Social Policy, 1950–1980.* New York: Basic Books.

National Academy of Sciences. Commission on Life Sciences. 1977. *Drinking Water and Health*, Vol. 1. New York: National Academy Press. (Accessed on-line at http://books.nap.edu)

National Board of Fire Underwriters. Committee of Twenty. 1905. *Report on the City of Savannah, GA.* New York: National Board of Fire Underwriters.

New York Times. Various issues, 1938.

North Carolina State Board of Health. *Biennial Report of the North Carolina State Board of Health to the General Assembly of North Carolina.* Raleigh: P. M. Hale State Printer and Binder. Various years.

Pittsburgh. The Pittsburgh Department (Board) of Public Health. *Annual Report of the Pittsburgh Department (Board) of Public Health.* Publisher unknown. Various years, 1888–1920.

Poppel, Frans van, and Cor van der Heijden. 1997. "The Effects of Water Supply on Infant and Childhood Mortality: A Review of Historical Evidence." *Health Transition Review*, 7: 113–48.

Poskitt, E. M. E., T. J. Cole, and R. G. Whitehead. 1999. "Less Diarrhoea but No Change in Growth: 15 Years' of Data from Three Gambian Villages." *Archives of Disease in Childhood*, 80: 115–20.

Preston, Samuel H., and Michael R. Haines. 1991. *Fatal Years: Child Mortality in Late Nineteenth Century America.* Princeton, N.J.: Princeton University Press.

Pritchett, Jonathan B., and İnsan Tunali. 1995. "Strangers' Disease: Determinants of Yellow Fever Mortality during the New Orleans Epidemic of 1853." *Explorations in Economic History*, 32: 517–39.

Rabinowitz, Howard N. 1978. *Race Relations in the Urban South, 1865–1890.* New York: Oxford University Press.

Roback, Jennifer. 1986. "The Political Economy of Segregation: The Case of Segregated Street Cars." *Journal of Economic History*, 46: 893–918.

Rosenberg, Charles E. 1962. *The Cholera Years, the United States in 1832, 1849, and 1866.* Chicago: University of Chicago Press.

Ruggles, S., and M. Sobek. 1997. *Integrated Public Use Microdata Series.* Minneapolis: Historical Census Projects, University of Minnesota.

Russell, James M. 1982. "Politics, Municipal Services, and the Working Class in Atlanta, 1865 to 1890." *Georgia Historical Quarterly*, 66: 467–91.

Russell, James M. 1988. *Atlanta, 1847–90: City Building in the Old South and the New.* Baton Rouge: Louisiana State University Press.

Savannah. 1901. *Report of the Hon. Herman Myers, Mayor, Together with the City Officers of the City of Savannah, GA., for the Year Ending December 31, 1900, and A History of the Municipal Government of Savannah from 1790 to 1901.* Compiled by Thomas Gamble, Jr., secretary to the Mayor.

Sedgwick, William T. 1922. *Principles of Sanitary Science and the Public Health, with Special Reference to the Causation and Prevention of Infectious Diseases.* New York: Macmillan.

Sedgwick, William T., and J. S. MacNutt. 1910. "On the Mills-Reincke Phenomenon and Hazen's Theorem Concerning the Decrease in Mortality from Diseases Other Than Typhoid Following the Purification of Public Water Supplies." *Journal of Infectious Diseases*, 7: 589–664.

Simon, Lawrence P. 1972. "Equal Protection in the Urban Environment: The Right to Equal Municipal Services." *Tulane Law Review*, 46: 498–525.

Slesnick, Daniel T. 1993. "Gaining Ground: Poverty in the Postwar United States." *Journal of Political Economy*, 101: 1–38.

Smith, Clarence E. 1919. "Role of the Sanitary Privy in the Control of Typhoid Fever." *American Journal of Public Health*, 12: 140–41.

Smith, Dale C. 1982. "The Rise and Fall of Typhomalarial Fever: II. Decline and Fall." *Journal of the History of Medicine and Allied Sciences*, 37: 287–321.

Stephens, Ina, and Myron Levine. 2002. "Management of Typhoid Fever in Children." *Pediatric Infectious Disease Journal*, 21: 157–59.

Szreter, Simon. 1988. "The Importance of Social Intervention in Britain's Mortality Decline c. 1850–1914: A Reinterpretation of the Role of Public Health." *Social History of Medicine*, 1: 1–37.

Szreter, Simon. 1997. "Economic Growth, Disruption, Deprivation, Disease, and Death: On the Importance of the Politics of Public Health for Development." *Population and Development Review*, 23: 693–728.

Taeuber, Karl E., and Alma F. Taeuber. 1965. *Negroes in Cities: Residential Segregation and Neighborhood Change.* Chicago: Aldine Press.

Tarr, Joel A. 1996. *The Search for the Ultimate Sink: Urban Pollution in Historical Perspective.* Akron, Ohio: University of Akron Press.

Teaford, Jon C. 1984. *The Unheralded Triumph: City Government in America, 1870–1900.* Baltimore: The Johns Hopkins University Press.

Tennessee State Board of Health. 1880. *First Report of the State Board of Health of the State of Tennessee, April, 1877 to October, 1880*. Nashville: Tavel and Howell, Printers to the State.

Terry, C. E. 1911. "Extermination of the House Fly in Cities, Its Necessity and Possibility." *American Journal of Public Health*, 2: 14–22.

Terry, C. E. 1912. "The Negro: His Relation to Public Health in the South." *American Journal of Public Health*, 3: 300–10.

Tolnay, Stewart E., and E. M. Beck. 1995. *A Festival of Violence: An Analysis of Southern Lynchings, 1882–1930*. Urbana: University of Illinois Press.

Tomes, Nancy. 1998. *The Gospel of Germs: Men, Women, and the Microbe in American Life*. Cambridge, Mass.: Harvard University Press.

Townsend, Joseph H. 1913. "Anti-Typhoid Vaccination." *American Journal of Public Health*, 3: 993–98.

Troesken, Werner. 1999. "Typhoid Rates and the Public Acquisition of Private Waterworks, 1880–1925." *Journal of Economic History*, 59: 927–48.

Troesken, Werner. 2001. "Race, Disease, and the Provision of Water in American Cities, 1889–1921." *Journal of Economic History*, 61: 750–76.

U.S. Bureau of the Census. *Census*. Various years, various volumes. Washington, D.C.: Government Printing Office.

U.S. Bureau of the Census. *General Statistics of Cities*. 1907, 1909 and 1915 volumes. Washington, D.C.: Government Printing Office.

U.S. Bureau of the Census. 1975. *Historical Statistics of the United States, Colonial Times to 1970, Parts 1 and 2*. Washington, D.C.: Government Printing Office.

U.S. Bureau of the Census. *Mortality Statistics*. Various years, 1900–1940. Washington, D.C.: Government Printing Office.

U.S. Bureau of the Census. *Social Statistics of Cities*. 1880 and 1890 volumes. Washington, D.C.: Government Printing Office.

U.S. Bureau of the Census. *Statistics of Cities*. 1903 and 1905 volumes. Washington, D.C.: Government Printing Office.

U.S. Department of Labor. 1897. "Condition of the Negro in Various Cities." *Bulletin of the Department of Labor*, No. 10. Washington, D.C.: Government Printing Office.

U.S. Department of Labor. Children's Bureau. 1917. *Infant Mortality: Results of a Field Study in Manchester, New Hampshire, Based on Births in One Year*. Infant Mortality Series, No. 6. Bureau Publication No. 20. Washington, D.C.: Government Printing Office.

U.S. Department of Labor. Children's Bureau. 1922. *Children of Preschool Age in Gary, Indiana*. Bureau Publication No. 122. Washington, D.C.: Government Printing Office.

U.S. Department of Labor. Children's Bureau. 1923. *Infant Mortality: Results of a Field Study in Baltimore, MD., Based on Births in One Year*. Bureau Publication No. 119. Washington, D.C.: Government Printing Office.

U.S. Public Health Service. *Annual Reports*. Various years.

Waring, George E. 1893. *Sewerage and Land Drainage*. New York: Van Nostrand.

Warner, Margaret. 1985. "Hunting the Yellow Fever Germ: The Principle and Practice of Etiological Proof in Late-Nineteenth Century America." *Bulletin of the History of Medicine*, 59: 361–82.

Warren, Christian. 1997. "Northern Chills, Southern Fevers: Race-Specific Mortality in American Cities, 1730–1900." *Journal of Southern History*, 63: 23–56.

Watson, Tara. 2002. "Public Health Investments and the Infant Mortality Gap: Evidence from Federal Sanitation Interventions and Hospitals on U.S. Indian Reservations." Unpublished paper. Department of Economics, Harvard University.

Whipple, George C. 1908. *Typhoid Fever: Its Causation, Transmission, and Prevention*. New York: Wiley.

White, Michael J. 1986. "Segregation and Diversity Measures in Population Distribution." *Population Index*, 52: 198–21.

Willis, John C. 2000. *Forgotten Time: The Yazoo-Mississippi Delta after the Civil War*. Charlottesville: University of Virginia Press.

Wing, Frank. 1914. "Thirty-Five Years of Typhoid: The Economic Cost to Pittsburgh and the Long Fight for Pure Water." In *The Pittsburgh District, Civic Frontage*, Paul Underwood Kellog, Ed., pp. 63–87. New York: Russell Sage Foundation. (Reprinted by Arno Press in 1974.)

Woodward, C. Vann. 1974. *The Strange Career of Jim Crow*. New York: Oxford University Press.

Wrenn, Lynette B. 1985. "The Memphis Sewer Experiment." *Tennessee Historical Quarterly*, 44: 337–49.

Wrenn, Lynette B. 1987. "The Impact of Yellow Fever on Memphis: A Reappraisal." *West Tennessee Historical Society Papers*, 41: 4–18.

Wright, Gavin. 1986. *Old South, New South: Revolutions in the Economic History of the South*. New York: Basic Books.

Wright, Gavin. 1999. "The Civil Rights Revolution as Economic History." *Journal of Economic History*, 59: 267–89.

Index